ADVANCES IN HEMODIAFILTRATION

Edited by **Ayman Karkar**

Advances in Hemodiafiltration
http://dx.doi.org/10.5772/61877
Edited by Ayman Karkar

Contributors

Aileen Grassmann, Bernard Canaud, Laura Scatizzi, Daniele Marcelli, David Johnson, Emily See, Carmel Hawley, John Agar, Sandip Mitra, Kunaal Kharbanda, Goran Imamović, Nusret Mehmedović, Caecilia Scholz, Vassilios Liakopoulos, Georgianos Panagiotis, Evangelia Dounousi, Theodoros Eleftheriadis, Abdulelah Essam A Nuqali, Luai Alhazmi, Mujeeb Sheikh, Ankush Moza, Samir H. Almueilo, Ayman Karkar, Khalid AlSaran

Published by InTech

Janeza Trdine 9, 51000 Rijeka, Croatia

Publishing Process Manager Dajana Pemac

Technical Editor SPi Global

Cover InTech Design team

First published September, 2016

Printed in Croatia

Additional hard copies can be obtained from orders@intechopen.com

Advances in Hemodiafiltration, Edited by Ayman Karkar

p. cm.

Print ISBN 978-953-51-2562-4

Online ISBN 978-953-51-2563-1

For EU product safety concerns:
IN TECH d.o.o., Prolaz Marije Krucifikse Kozulić 3, 51000 Rijeka, Croatia,
info@intechopen.com or visit our website at intechopen.com.

Meet the editor

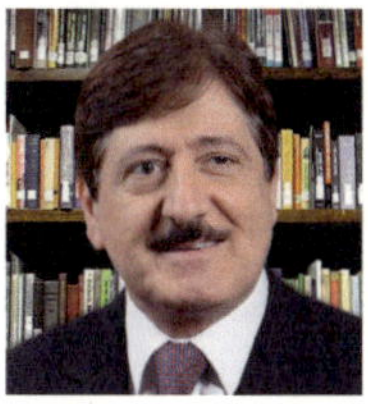

Following his graduation from the medical school, Dr. Ayman Karkar received his MSc degree in Nephrology and Hypertension and PhD degree in Renal Medicine from the Hammersmith Hospital, University of London. Dr. Karkar is a consultant physician and nephrologist and Fellow of the Royal College of Physicians (FRCP) of London, Edinburgh, Glasgow, and Ireland, and Fellow of the American National Kidney Foundation (FNKF) and the American Society of Nephrology (FASN). He has authored several books and published over 140 articles and abstracts in peer-reviewed medical journals. Dr. Karkar is currently a consultant physician and nephrologist at the Ministry of Health, Saudi Arabia.

Contents

Preface

Hemodialysis (HD) treatment had over many years improved the survival rate of patients with end-stage renal disease (ESRD). However, standard or conventional HD prescription is far from being optimal in replacing the function of normal kidneys. Its unphysiologic clearance pattern and inability to remove all types and sizes of uremic toxins result in inter- and intra-dialysis complications and unacceptable high rates of cardiovascular morbidity and mortality. Hemodiafiltration (HDF), which had attracted much attention in recent years as an optimum modality of HD, offers the most physiologic clearance profile for a broad range of small-, medium-, and large-sized toxic molecules. Implementation of HDF can result in quality care achievements in clinical practice and reduction in morbidity and mortality rates among HD patients. This *Advances in Hemodiafiltration* book, with its wide coverage of various aspects of HDF, can be considered as a guide to the daily practice and how best possible medical outcomes can be achieved in dialysis patients. The tremendous efforts and valued contributions of all participating authors are much appreciated.

Finally, my special thanks and appreciation go to the Publishing Process Manager, Ms. Dajana Pemac, for her great organization efforts and professional assistance.

Ayman Karkar
consultant physician and nephrologist
Ministry of Health, Saudi Arabia

Chapter 1

Introductory Chapter

Ayman Karkar

Additional information is available at the end of the chapter

http://dx.doi.org/10.5772/64607

Conventional hemodialysis (CHD) treatment is a basic renal replacement therapy (RRT) that has been serving and supporting the life of patients with end-stage renal disease (ESRD) for many years. The capabilities of this modality, which is based on the physiologic principle of diffusion, are however limited. In reality, CHD can remove excess fluids but with some difficulty in maintaining hemodynamic stability and can only clear small-size uremic toxins of less than 500 Da such as urea and creatinine but not larger-size uremic toxins of more than 500 Da. These include middle molecules such as β2-microglobulin and protein-bound molecules such as indoxyl sulfate and *p*-cresol, where their accumulation in the blood can lead to hemodialysis-related amyloidosis and endothelial inflammation and toxicity, respectively. This may explain, at least in part, the high incidence of morbidity and mortality in patients treated with CHD. Furthermore, the intradialytic complications and post-dialysis tiredness, fatigue, and exhaustion have negatively influenced the quality of life of dialysis patients.

The recent technical advances in dialysis machine specifications, production of ultrapure water by modern water treatment system, innovation of synthetic biocompatible high-cut-off membranes, achievement of scientific knowledge in implementing the other physiologic principle of convection, and combining diffusion with convection have all revolutionized the dialysis technique. For example, the modality of hemofiltration (HF), which is based on convection, is capable of removing larger-size molecules of more than 500 Da, whereas the modality of hemodiafiltration (HDF), which combines diffusion and convection, is capable of removing small- and larger-size uremic toxins. In addition, both of these techniques provide more hemodynamic stability, which is more evident with online HDF. Over many years, multiple observational and randomized clinical trials showed plenty of clinical benefits of online HDF, which had significant impact on morbidity and mortality rates. Since the establishment and implementation of online HDF, a significant experience and knowledge have been gained in ways of its application and achievement of beneficial clinical results (**Figure 1**).

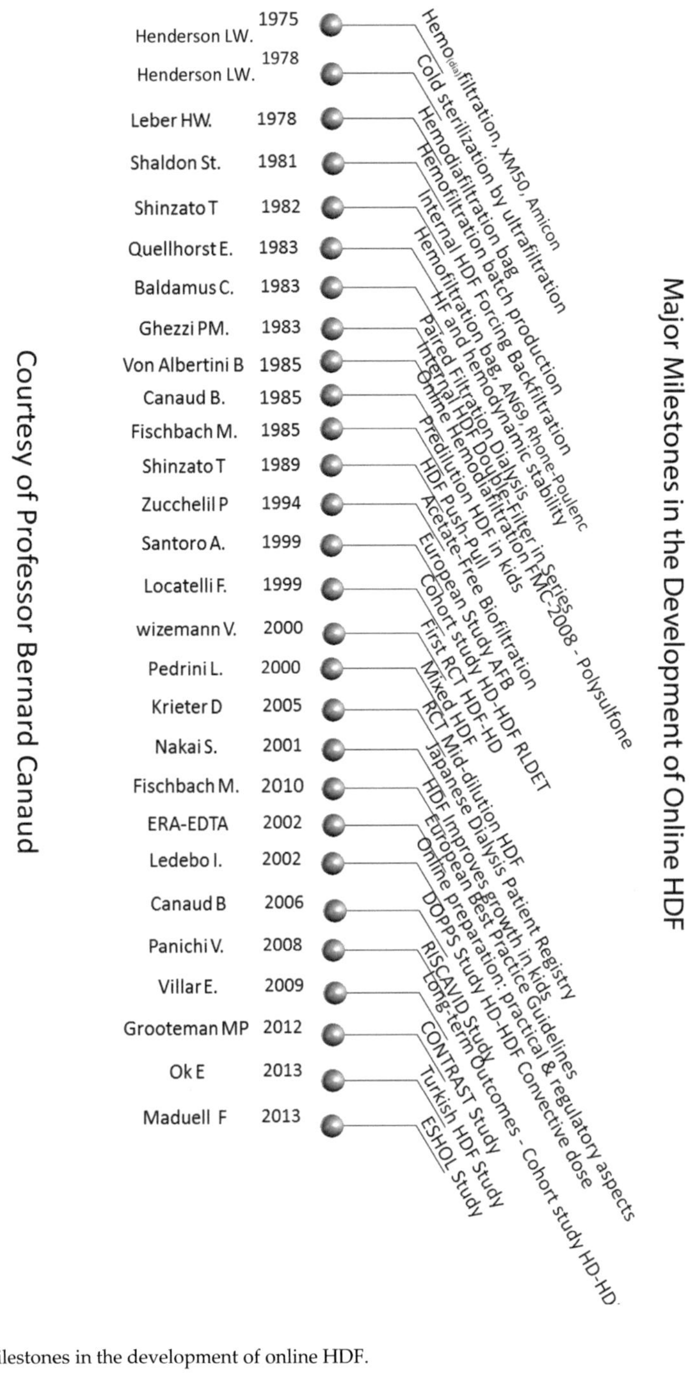

Figure 1. Major milestones in the development of online HDF.

The *Advances in Hemodiafiltration* book has been specifically designed to describe and demonstrate the treatment modality of HDF from its basic concepts to the most recent advances in the techniques of its implementation. Under specific titles of specially created chapters, this

http://dx.doi.org/10.5772/64607

book covers principles of HDF, generation of ultrapure water, fluid convection and reinfusion, factors affecting convective dose, dialysis machine-dependent technical factors, prescription of HDF, performance and effectiveness of HDF, clinical benefits including results of major randomized clinical trials, effects of online HDF on arterial stiffness and heart failure, quality of life of patients on HDF, cost-effectiveness of HDF, and applicability of HDF at home.

Author details

Karkar Ayman

Address all correspondence to: aymankarkar@yahoo.com

Ministry of Health, Riyadh, Saudi Arabia

Chapter 2

Principles of Haemodiafiltration: Rationale for Improved Patients' Survival

Goran Imamović, Bernard Canaud,
Nusret Mehmedović and Cäcilia Scholz

Additional information is available at the end of the chapter

http://dx.doi.org/10.5772/63067

Abstract

Haemodiafiltration (HDF) is a renal replacement modality that combines diffusion and enhanced convection in order to remove small- and middle-molecular-weight compounds, respectively. They are removed along solvent drag effect of ultrafiltration through increased transmembrane pressure (TMP), whereas the replacement solution is infused intravenously at equal amount minus the desired fluid volume removal for achieving dry weight. Limiting factors for high-volume on-line haemodiafiltration (HV oHDF) are blood flow and viscosity (haematocrit, protocrit), filter performance and technical features of HDF monitor. Most recent advanced technology of dynamic analysis of pressure pulses along the blood flow pathway in the dialyser has enabled optimal ultrafiltration flow performances. HV oHDF offers today the best compromise of cardioprotective option by reducing cardiovascular risk factors in end-stage kidney disease patients. Recent randomised controlled trials (RCTs), individual participant data meta-analyses and a number of observational studies have shown the evidence of survival advantage of HDF over conventional haemodialysis (HD). The convective volume has become the key quantifier for HV oHDF as the measure of dialysis dose. Its cut-off values for better survival have been recognised, but the research is still needed in the years to come to set the required optimal volumes tailored to individual patients' needs.

Keywords: haemodialysis, haemodiafiltration, convection, ultrafiltration, mortality

1. Introduction

The uremic syndrome is characterised by an accumulation of uremic toxins due to inadequate kidney function. There have been more than 90 compounds considered to be uremic toxins listed by the European Uremic Toxin Work Group. Sixty-eight have a molecular weight less than 500 Da, 10 have a molecular weight between 500 and 12,000 Da and 12 exceed 12,000 Da. Twenty-five solutes (28%) are protein bound [1]. These figures are further increasing with the adoption of new knowledge and technology of uremic toxins detection.

The clearance of solutes during conventional haemodialysis (HD) depends on their size and the concentration gradient across the dialysis membrane. Solutes weighing less than 500 Da are considered low-molecular-weight solutes and they are removed by passive diffusion down a favourable concentration gradient. Urea is considered a marker of such toxins. Its clearance, as measured by Kt/Vurea, correlates with patient morbidity [2] showing the evidence that such toxins contribute to the uremic syndrome.

However, despite improvements in technology and patient care, the mortality rate of patients on maintenance dialysis remains high, at approximately 15–20% per year [3]. As specified in the United States Renal Data System report, the expected remaining life span after the initiation of renal replacement therapy was eight years for dialysis patients aged 40–44 and 4.5 years for those 60–64 years of age. In general population the ranges of the expected remaining life span at specified ages are 30–40 years and 17–22 years, respectively. The values in older dialysis patients are only slightly better than those in patients with lung cancer [4]. Therefore, there is an obvious need to change the practices and to attempt to approach the problem differently.

2. Historic background

In an attempt to reduce mortality, it was postulated in 1983 that a higher Kt/V than commonly prescribed during conventional short dialysis may increase survival among patients undergoing renal replacement therapies [5]. However, the hemodialysis (HEMO) study failed to show a positive effect on patient survival when dialysis dose per haemodialysis session was increased above the current K/DOQI recommendations [6]. Possible explanation for this unfavourable outcome could be in the kinetics of urea removal which is representative of small solutes, but not of larger sized molecules such as middle molecules, large-molecular-weight proteins or protein-bound solutes, thereby making Kt/V misleading. Clearance of urea accounts for only one-sixth of physiological clearance [1]. In addition, several shortcomings are associated with short dialysis schedules that are not captured by Kt/V index such as extracellular fluid volume control, phosphate control and adequate removal of middle and larger uremic molecules compounds.

Beta-2 microglobulin levels are associated with the development of dialysis-related amyloidosis and possibly reduced survival [7]. It seems likely that beta-2 microglobulin is a marker for overall middle-molecule clearance, including more toxic and as yet unidentified uremic compounds [8–11]. Those solutes are better removed by high-flux membranes compared to low-flux membranes due to their more porous characteristics with increased permeability.

Whether survival differs upon exposure to randomly assigned high- or low-flux membranes was also evaluated in the HEMO study [6]. No difference was observed. The same result was obtained in the Membrane Permeability Outcome study, in which patients were also randomly assigned to high- or low-flux dialysis membranes [12].

In an attempt to improve patients' outcomes, alternative renal replacement therapies have been developed, since removal by diffusion becomes less efficient as the molecular weight of a solute increases. Therefore, the need to mimic the kidney function seems to become mandatory in order to enhance middle-molecule removal because the diffusion in the tubules and loop of Henle follows filtration in glomerulus, which is the principle of convection (**Figure 1**).

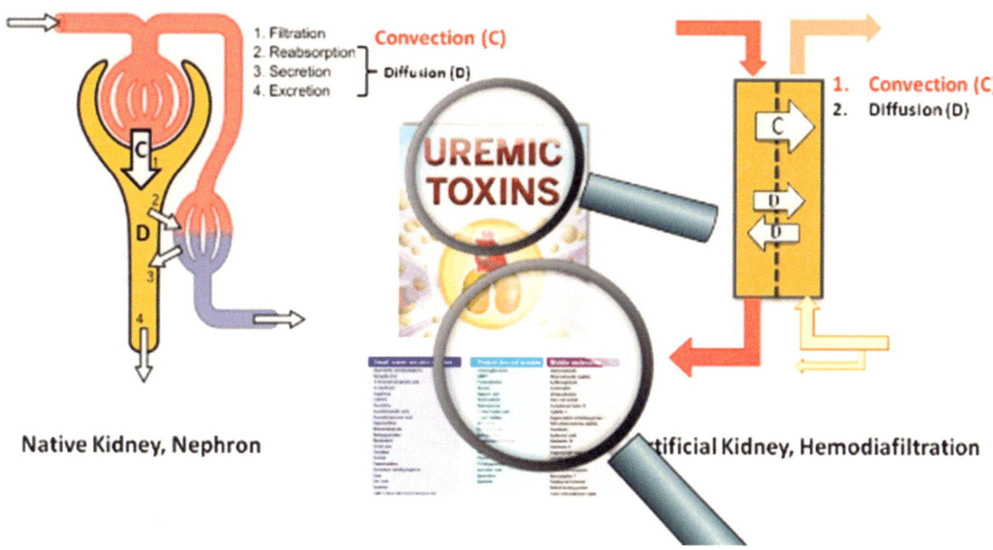

Figure 1. Mimicking native kidney function to enhance middle-molecule removal.

Haemofiltration (HF) is the treatment modality that employs convection in order to facilitate removal of larger molecular weight solutes while using high-flux dialysers only. In convection the small- and large-molecular-weight solutes are removed in the ultrafiltrate by solvent drag. Although HF is effective in the removal of the larger molecular weight solutes, it is less effective in the removal of small molecules as it is restricted by the magnitude of the ultrafiltration volume achievable. Haemodiafiltration (HDF) is the treatment modality that combines diffusion and enhanced convection in order to facilitate removal of small-molecular-weight solutes. Moreover, small-molecule removal is further increased with the use of high-volume on-line HDF (HV oHDF) (see section "Towards more cardioprotective renal replacement therapy") and can be higher than haemodialysis, depending upon the volume of the replacement solution [13].

The ratio between treatment techniques, processes and molecular weights of the solutes is shown in **Figure 2**.

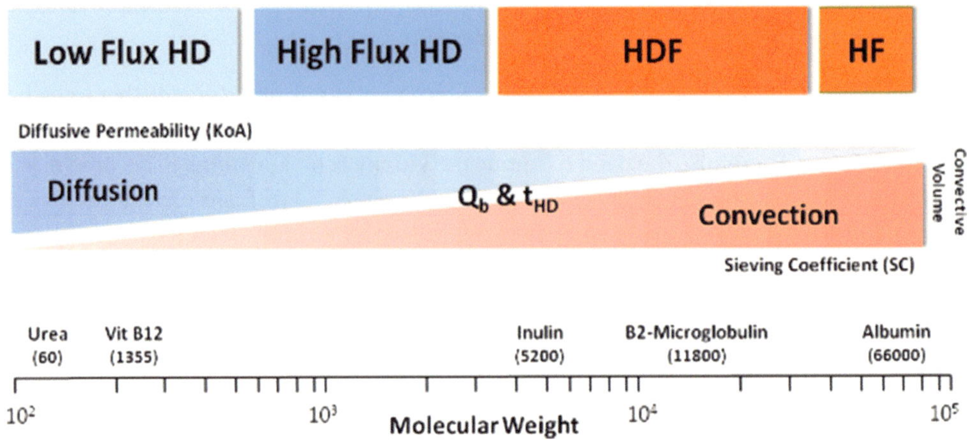

Figure 2. The ratio between treatment techniques, processes and molecular weights of solutes. HD, haemodialysis; HDF, haemodiafiltration; HF, haemofiltration; KoA, mass transfer area coefficient; Q_B, blood flow; t_{HD}, duration of HD session; SC, sieving coefficient (the proportion of a substance to be removed for a particular filter).

The utilization of convective therapies has been variable. Between 1998 and 2001, about 12% of patients were on HDF in the European countries participating in the Dialysis Outcome and Practice Patterns Study (DOPPS) study [14].

There have not been too many studies to compare the patients' survival between convective modalities and high-flux HD. One of them was Italian MAMHEBI study, which was a randomised controlled trial (RCT). Significantly higher three-year survival was noted with HF (68% versus 52%) [15]. Dialysis Outcome and Practice Patterns Study (DOPPS) was prospective observational study which showed better survival with HDF, but it compared high-efficiency HDF with composite predictor of high- and low-flux haemodialysis [14]. Vilar et al. conducted retrospective cohort study and showed better survival with on-line HDF than with high-flux haemodialysis [16], as well as Imamović et al. in incident patients' population [17], but the latter three were epidemiological studies and RCT to show survival benefit of HDF over conventional HD was still missing.

3. Technological principles of haemodiafiltration

Ultrafiltrate volume, derived from Q_{UF} times treatment time (**Figure 3**), is removed by the dialysis machine through increased transmembrane pressure (TMP), whereas the replacement solution is infused intravenously at equal volume minus the desired fluid volume removal to preserve extracellular fluid balance and isovolemic state. The replaced solution represents *substitution volume*, whereas convective volume represents the sum of substitution volume and desired fluid volume removal during the dialysis session.

Filtration fraction (FF) (proportion of ultrafiltration volume obtained compared with total blood volume processed during the HD session) was traditionally supposed to be 25% (**Figure 3**).

http://dx.doi.org/10.5772/63067

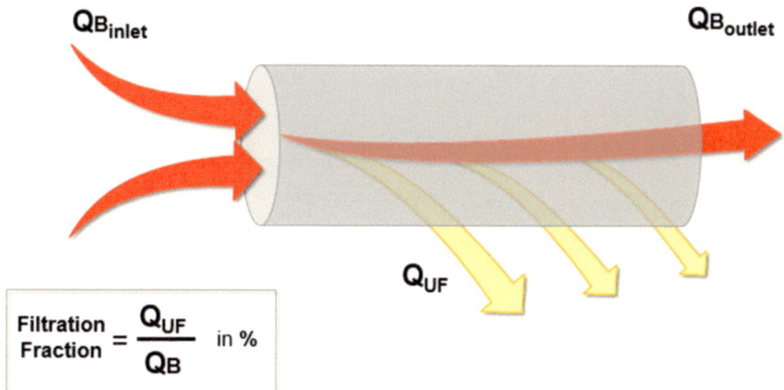

Figure 3. Filtration fraction. Q_B, blood flow rate; Q_{UF}, ultrafiltration flow rate.

3.1. Dilution modes

The fluid can be substituted either after the dialyser as the reference mode (post-dilution mode) or before the dialyser (pre-dilution mode) (**Figure 4**), or both (mixed dilution mode).

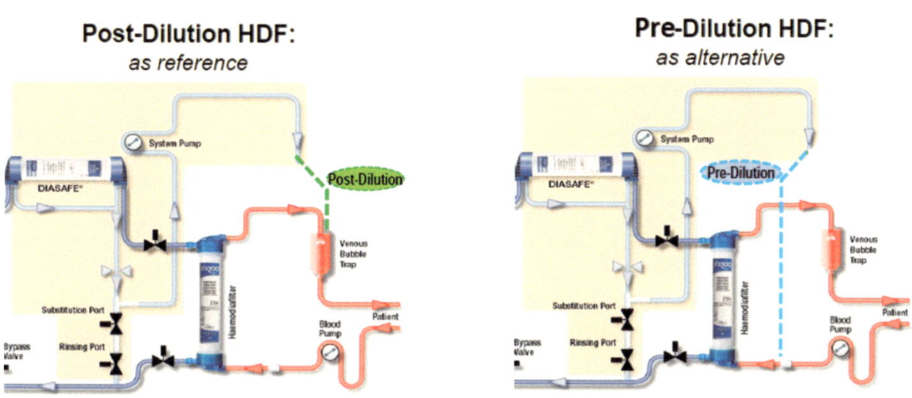

Figure 4. Dilution modes in haemodiafiltration; HDF, haemodiafiltration.

Choice on which dilution mode to apply depends on patient haemorheology and clinical performance (**Table 1**).

Post-dilution HDF	Pre-dilution HDF	Mixed-dilution HDF
Pros	**Pros**	**Pros**
High solute clearance and removal	Haemodilution	Avoids the drawbacks of post- and pre-modes
Reduced consumption of substitution volume	Decreased viscosity and oncotic pressure	**Cons**

Post-dilution HDF	Pre-dilution HDF	Mixed-dilution HDF
Cons	Reduced fibres and membrane fouling	Requires specific hardware equipment and software
Haemoconcentration	Preserved hydraulic and solute membrane permeability	
Increased viscosity and oncotic pressure	Reduced membrane stress	
Fibres and membrane fouling	**Cons**	
Reduced hydraulic and solute membrane permeability	Reduced solute clearance and removal	
Increased transmembrane pressure	Increased consumption of substitution volume	
Reduced sieving coefficient		
Fibre clotting		
Potential alarms		
Increasing membrane stress		
Potential albumin leakage		

HDF – Haemodiafiltration

Table 1. Pros and cons of dilution modes.

4. Water for dialysis

Possible pyrogenic reactions were considerable threat to patients on HDF since the risk of microbiological contamination with high substitution volumes was increased. Besides, costs were greater with increased substitution volumes used as well as with storage bags for them. Therefore, the need for the production of high purity substitution fluid at lower cost was a challenge, not only because of threatening pyrogenic reactions and financial constraints but also because of higher risk of accelerated atherosclerosis and malnutrition due to ongoing low-grade inflammation [18]. Therefore, the American Association for the Advancement of Medical Instrumentation set the microbiological standards for water for dialysis at <200 colony-forming units (CFU) and <0.5 endotoxin units (EU)/ml. The European Pharmacopoeia was more stringent with <100 CFU and <0.25 EU/ml. Eventually, <0.1 CFU and <0.03 EU/ml were adopted for a solution to be considered "ultra-pure" and it is now widely used even for conventional haemodialysis [19].

"On-line" fluid production has enabled the concept of on-line HDF (oHDF). It facilitates the provision of an unlimited volume of sterile, non-pyrogenic substitution fluid not requiring storage, which is an efficient approach to prevent bacterial contamination and growth at a cost close to that of dialysate for conventional haemodialysis [20, 21]. The first step of the process includes the filtration of the water after it is produced using the reverse osmosis technique. The water is then used for the production of dialysate. This step has also been adopted in several haemodialysis machines to produce dialysate of improved purity. The second step includes further filtration of the dialysate. Finally, a third filtration by a disposable microfilter completes the creation of the substitution solution. The disposable microfilter is replaced at the end of the dialysis session. The dialysate prior to the last filtration is used for the diffusive element of HDF. The purity achieved using this approach has been repeatedly confirmed [21, 22] (**Figure 5**).

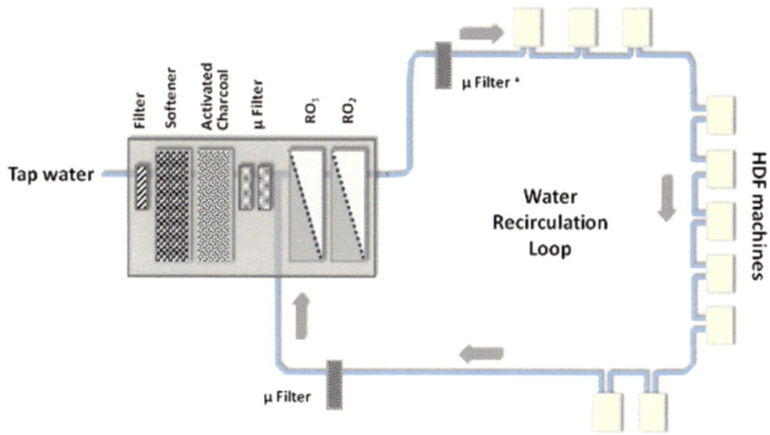

Figure 5. One of the examples of water treatment system in the dialysis centre in Hemodialysis Unit of Lapeyronie Hospital in Montpellier (France) with microfilters depicted plus two microfilters within HDF machines (not depicted) showing the water for dialysis passing through HDF machines. The amount used ends up in the sewage; RO, reverse osmosis; HDF, haemodiafiltration.

So, an additional step to ensure full safety of dialysis and substitution fluids is to implement two sterilising ultrafilters built in within HDF machines on the path after the dialysate was prepared. They are disinfected regularly with the HDF machine and are replaced after a certain time of use as defined by manufacturer.

From an economic perspective, the added cost of the ultrafilters used to prepare the substitution solution has been nullified because of growing tendency of using ultra-pure dialysate even in conventional haemodialysis, thereby leaving the only difference in cost in the amount of water consumed per treatment. Above all, the remaining cost has been balanced by the biochemical and clinical benefits of HDF [20].

5. Rational for improved patients' survival on high-volume haemodiafiltration

The European Dialysis Working Group (EUDIAL) performed a systematic review and meta-analysis of randomised controlled trials on haemodiafiltration in 2014 and found the beneficial effect of post-dilution oHDF over HD in reducing all-cause and cardiovascular mortality (pooled RR-0.84; 95% CI, 0.73–0.96) and recommended wide acceptance of this treatment modality [23]. EUDIAL recommends the adoption of effective convective volume as a key quantifier for HDF. Providing time is constant and anticoagulation is adequate, limiting factors for high-volume haemodiafiltration (i.e. the amount of substitution fluid produced) are blood viscosity, filter performance and blood flow rate.

5.1. Limiting factors for high-volume on-line haemodiafiltration

5.1.1. Blood viscosity as a limiting factor for high-volume on-line haemodiafiltration

It is not only that FF from **Figure 3** accounts for the proportion of UF volume in the blood volume, but in reality, FF is even higher, because UF volume comes from plasma water, not from the whole blood. **Figure 6** shows the example of a patient with FF of 0.30 (UF rate 120 ml/min and blood flow rate 400 ml/min). However, if the haematocrit of this patient is 30%, it means that his/her plasma water flow is only 280 ml/min, which increases FF to 0.43 (**Figure 6**).

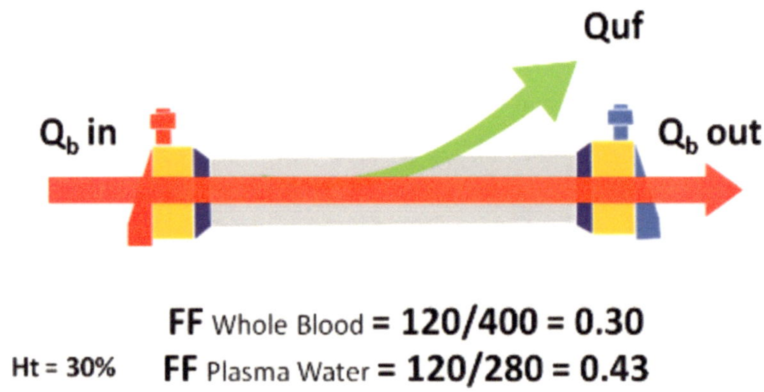

Figure 6. Increased filtration fraction in plasma water.

Consequently, too much convective volume increases the risk of haemoconcentration, thereby compromising the fine balance between the two by interfering with membrane permeability both on hydraulic and solute fluxes.

5.1.2. Filter performance as a limiting factor for high-volume on-line haemodiafiltration

The efficiency of HDF might be improved by increasing the size of the surface area of the membranes (provided optimal blood flow was achieved), so that high efficiency might be achieved with a surface area of 2.2 m^2, as opposed to the standard surface of 1.4 m^2, thereby allowing much more substitution fluid to be replaced at a rate of 120 ml/min in post-dilution mode, in contrast to 60 ml/min which was achieved with standard surface [24].

The size of a membrane pore dictates the sieving coefficient (SC) of a substance to be removed. The higher the sc, the higher the UF and clearance of a particular solute. The reduction ratios of beta-2 microglobulin with low-flux, high-flux haemodialysis and HDF are 20, 60 and 75% per session, respectively [25]. The EUDIAL group, nominated by the European Renal Association – European Dialysis and Transplant Association (ERA–EDTA), set the SC for beta-2 microglobulin at minimum of 0.6 [26] in high-flux filters (which are mandatory with HDF). However, in order to achieve the optimal outcome for the patients, filters are nowadays designed with even higher SC for beta-2 microglobulin of 0.8 for efficient elimination, but still retention of albumin (**Figure 7**).

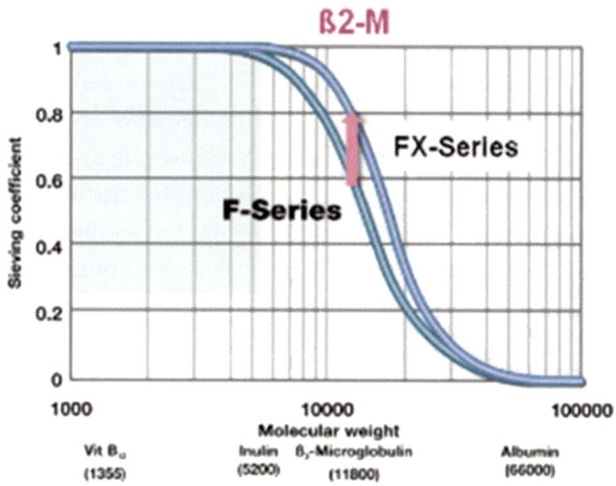

Figure 7. Solute membrane permeability: higher sieving coefficient for beta-2 microglobulin.

Correlation between ultrafiltered volume and beta-2 microglobulin elimination is linear, as specified by Lornoy et al. (**Figure 8**) [27].

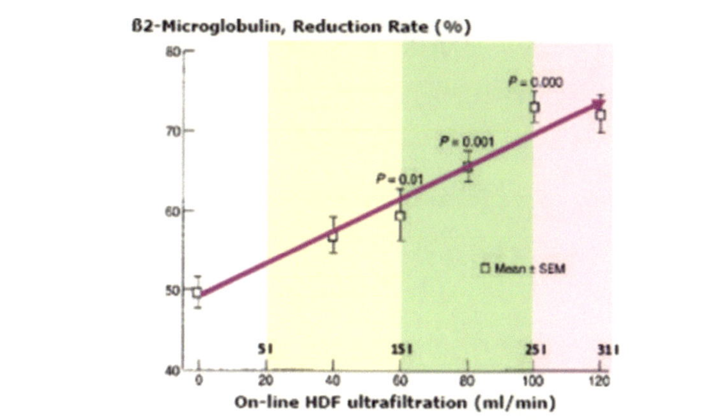

Figure 8. A linear function of ultrafiltered volume and beta-2 microglobulin elimination. HDF, haemodiafiltration (with permission of authors).

Enhanced clearances of middle molecules such as beta-2 microglobulin [28] and phosphate [29] and other small molecules, such as homocysteine and complement D factor [30] are the main biochemical benefits of convective-based treatment over conventional HD.

5.1.3. Blood flow as a limiting factor for high-volume haemodiafiltration

On-line monitoring of blood parameters allows adjustment of ultrafiltration rate to identify the patient-specific exchange rate possible at any given point in time while enabling haemodynamic stability. The substitution rate is adjusted to blood flow rate, thereby controlling haemoconcentration, whereas blood flow rate is adjusted to dialysis flow rate to control diffusion [31] (as for the diffusion component on-line clearance monitoring is used and the goal is to achieve spKt/V of 1.4). Therefore, if the blood flow rate drops from 100 L to 70 L per session, and the total UF volume remains at 25 L, the filtration fraction rises from 25% to 37% (**Figure 9**), which may generate a lot of difficulty during the session, lot of alarms and lot of critical TMP notifications, and the session may not end with a volume that was targeted.

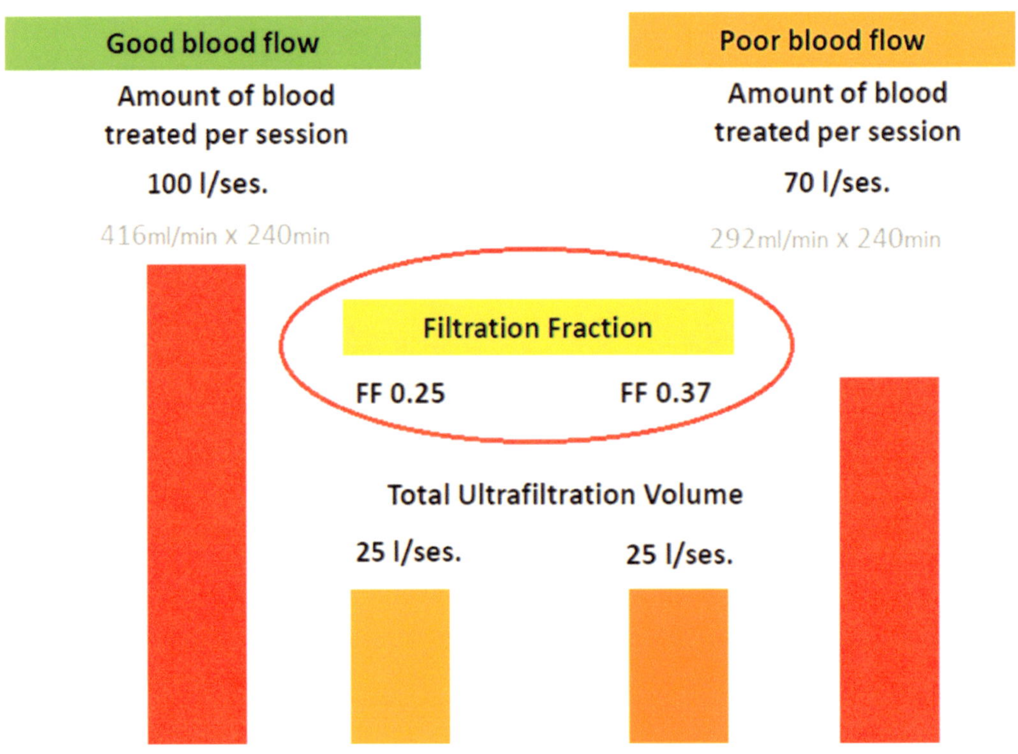

Figure 9. The impact of blood flow on filtration fraction.

6. Towards more cardioprotective renal replacement therapy

In the very beginning of oHDF era, both the physician and the nurse in charge were supposed to do manual interventions in an attempt to prescribe and to keep the desired convective volume for each individual patient, respectively. The physician was able to do manual calculation based on the formula that included optimal blood flow rate, desired ultrafiltration rate to compensate for interdialytic weight gain, haematocrit, total proteins and filter performance, which was frequently producing alarms indicating threatening haemoconcentration and possible membrane fouling due to an excessive ultrafiltration rate. Therefore, the nurse had to carefully monitor the TMP (indicator of threatening problems) and react during the session in three possible ways in order to prevent TMP from reaching critical level: (a) rinse the dialyser with substitution fluid or normal saline, (b) decrease the UF rate or (c) switch to conventional haemodialysis. The latter two interventions were reducing the anticipated convective volume in the dialysis prescription, whereas the former intervention was only temporarily fixing the problem.

The advanced technology of automatic adaptation by the built-in software AutoSub®, Fresenius Medical Care or Ultracontrol®, Baxter, was later developed in order to achieve alarm-free setting and to avoid the related problems, so that no manual calculation was needed any more by the physician in charge, but yet not all parameters with impact on flow conditions and blood viscosity were considered in formula. Therefore a nurse still had to do manual interventions because warning notification used to be received by the built-in software in order to opt for (a) ignoring the warning; (b) accepting the warning and letting the software reduce the UF at a new recommended rate in order to be within a safe range and prevent TMP from reaching critical level, albeit reducing the expected convective volume defined at the beginning of the session; or (c) turning off software monitoring. Besides, the nurse can always turn off the substitution pump and switch to HD.

Finally, with the development of the new technology for automatic ultrafiltration control in the dialyser, alarm-free maximisation of substitution volumes has been achieved, which is based not only on information about conditions across the membrane but also along the blood flow pathway in the dialyser, so that calculation of substitution volume based on the parameters specified above has become obsolete [32]. This was shown in a crossover study of patients treated during 240-min sessions on the same day with three different blood flow rates (Q_B300, Q_B350 and Q_B380) and switched after two consecutive weeks from conventional HDF to this new technology. The convective volumes were 24.8 ± 3.1, 27.8 ± 3.0, 28.8 ± 2.4 and 23.9 ± 1.2, 27.2 ± 1.9, 28.5 ± 2.1, respectively ($p > 0.05$), to provide the evidence that the biological markers specified above are not needed for each and every haemodialysis session in order to achieve optimisation of the procedure [33].

This innovative technology is known as AutoSub plus mode [32] (**Figure 10**).

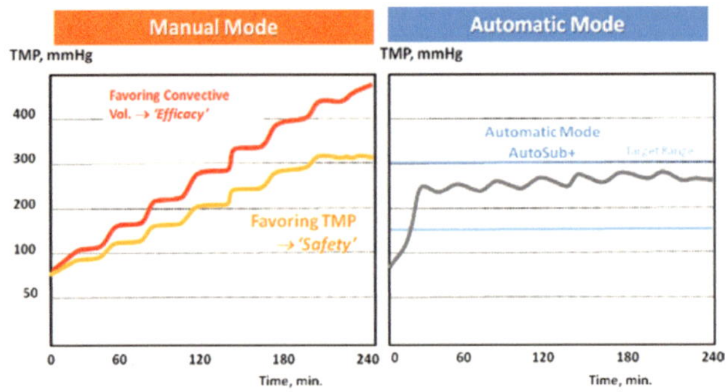

Figure 10. Switch from manual to automatic mode. TMP, transmembrane pressure.

Figure 10 shows the red line in manual mode favouring increasing convective volume and efficacy, whereas yellow line represents safety and favours TMP limitations, which means that TMP increases over time during the dialysis session as convective volume increases. However, in automatic mode on the right side of **Figure 10**, the optimisation of substitution volume has been achieved by setting the safety target range so that the machine itself sets the safe TMP target range and continuously regulates the optimal UF rate at an optimal time throughout the session in order to keep the TMP in optimal range to prevent haemoconcentration and membrane complications specified above (**Table 1**). However, the nurse can still switch to manual mode or even to conventional HD should extraordinary conditions prevent high-volume oHDF (such as special rheologic properties of a patient's blood) [32]. Owing to continuous analysis of haemorheological conditions throughout the dialysis session, continuous adaptation of UF flow takes place (**Figure 11**).

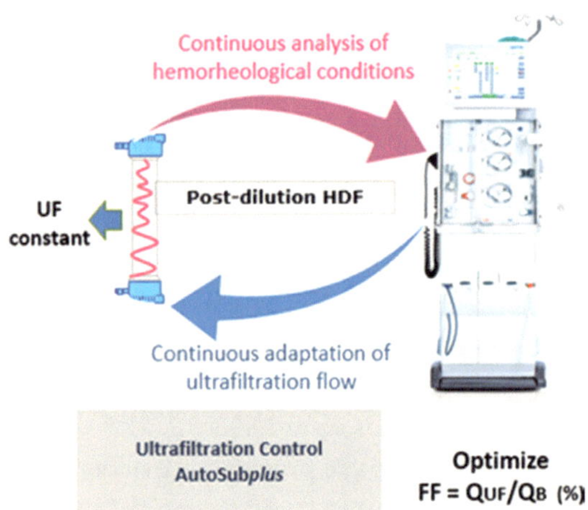

Figure 11. Continuous adaptation of ultrafiltration flow in AutoSub plus mode while keeping UF loss constant; red line within the dialyser illustrates dynamic analysis of pressure pulses along the blood flow pathway; UF, ultrafiltrate to be lost during the dialysis session; HDF, haemodiafiltration; FF, filtration fraction; Q_{UF}, ultrafiltrate flow; Q_B, blood flow.

http://dx.doi.org/10.5772/63067

For this improvement sieving coefficient for beta-2 microglobulin was further increased to 0.9 in a new series of Cordiax© dialysers (**Figure 12**).

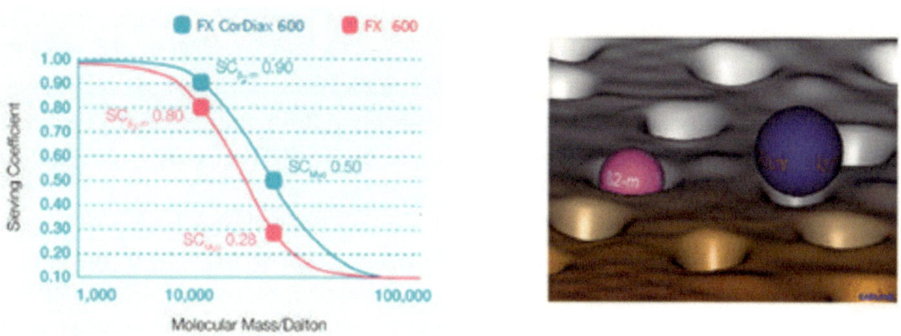

Figure 12. New series of Cordiax© dialysers with sieving coefficient for beta-2 microglobulin of 0.9 achieved by widened pore diameter which permits better molecule removal, but still retention of albumin (simplified graph based on manufacturer's internal data).

The result is the improved removal of middle molecules (while ensuring the retention of albumin) due to increased filtration fraction, thereby generating increased substitution fluid volumes, with no need to even keep the high blood flow rate, so that equally adequate dialysis can also be delivered to patients with suboptimal blood flow rates (such as inpatients with poor vascular access or inadequate needle size). This technology introduced the concept of high-volume oHDF with substitution volumes >20 L as well as the related concept of cardioprotective haemodialysis due to its beneficial effects of cardiovascular system. It introduced the new era of high-volume cardioprotective renal replacement therapy as the major clinical effect of high-volume oHDF.

7. Clinical effects of high-volume oHDF

The main clinical effects of high-volume oHDF include haemodynamic stability [34, 35], possibly improved quality of life [30], a delay in the development of dialysis-related amyloidosis [36], improvement in anaemia management [17], plasma lipid profiles [37] and inflammation [37].

Haemodynamic stability is maintained by salt loading via substitution fluid administration [38]. A higher predialysis plasma sodium concentration in patients with higher frequency of oHDF was reported, thus suggesting reduced sodium removal [39]. Haemodynamic stability is maintained by decreasing core body temperature as a result of the infusion of large amounts of fluid at a lower temperature, leading to vasoconstriction [34]. Imamović et al. demonstrated reduction in both erythropoietin (EPO) consumption and EPO resistance index in patients on HV oHDF compared to high-flux HD [17], which reveals the evidence of an increased haemodynamic stability due to improved anaemia management [40].

8. The impact of substitution volume in haemodiafiltration on patients' survival

In the era of convective treatment modalities employed in oHDF, the substitution volume appears to be critical for patient survival in prevalent patients [14, 41–43]. The Dialysis Outcomes and Practice Patterns Study (DOPPS) showed better survival of prevalent patients with high-volume HDF defined as having a substitution fluid volume of >15 L compared to low-flux HD (RR 0.65) [14]. The Turkish RCT and the CONTRAST RCT revealed survival benefits of oHDF over conventional HD in prevalent patients with 17.4 L (RR 0.54) and 21.95 L (RR 0.61) of substitution and convective volumes, respectively, but only in post hoc analyses [41, 42]. The first positive RCT in favour of improved survival of oHDF over conventional HD was the ESHOL study which showed convective volumes cut-offs of 23.1–25.4 L (RR 0.60) and >25.4 L (RR 0.55) in the intermediate and upper tertiles, respectively, also in post hoc analysis of prevalent patients' data [43]. Eventually, the observational Balkan study in incident HD patients conducted in Bosnia and Herzegovina, Serbia and Slovenia, while using European Clinical Database (EuCliD®), [17] showed the lowest RR for mortality of 0.29 on high-volume oHDF compared to high-flux conventional HD. The substitution volume cut-off of 20.4 L was discriminating between low- and high-volume oHDF, which makes the convective volume at least in the range of the one achieved in ESHOL study. Consequently, overall negative correlation may be observed between increasing ultrafiltration volumes and mortality risks in patients on convective-based treatments in comparison with conventional HD. **Figure 13** shows descriptive hazard ratios for mortality based on literature data (not on forest-plot analysis).

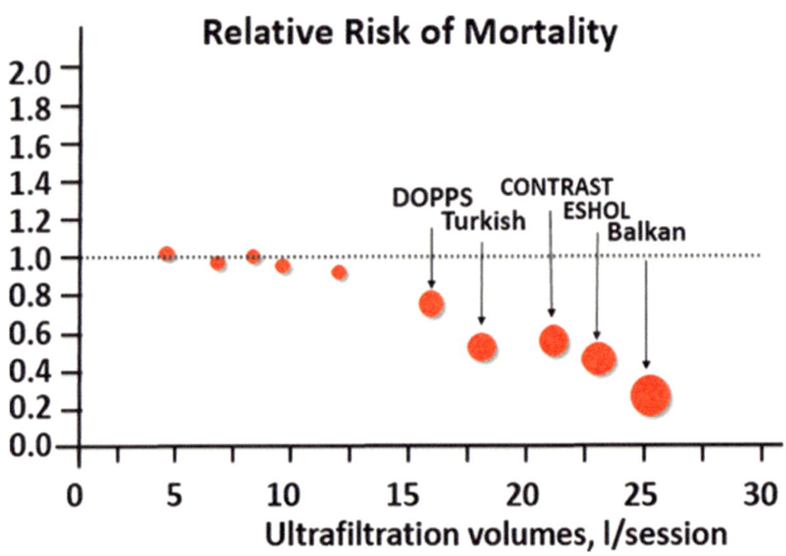

Figure 13. Negative correlation between increasing ultrafiltration volumes and decreasing relative risk of mortality in patients on haemodiafiltration.

http://dx.doi.org/10.5772/63067

Recently, Canaud et al. aimed at determining optimal convection volume in 2293 international incident dialysis patients treated for 4 h with oHDF in post-dilution mode. Two-year survival rate was found to increase at about 55 L of convection volume per week and to stay increased up to about 75 L/week [44].

9. Conclusions

HV oHDF is a renal replacement treatment modality that is becoming increasingly employed in haemodialysis units worldwide because of a strong body of evidence of its survival benefit over conventional haemodialysis. Optimal substitution volume has become the measure of convective dose, reflecting mainly middle- and large-molecular-weight solutes, and it completed former Kt/V that was mainly dedicated to small-molecular-weight solutes. Both dialysis dose components are intent to act synergistically and provide more precise tools for assessing dialysis adequacy. More specifically, convective dose should be tailored to individual patients' needs depending on optimal blood flow rate, rheological blood conditions and the condition of vascular access. Studies in this field are still needed to set the cut-offs of substitution volumes to be adjusted based on the residual renal function. An alternative proposal for dialysis dose is serum beta-2 microglobulin clearance or plasma level determination, but those measurements are relatively expensive and confounded by calibration differences and variations in the generation rate. The convective volume must be set for each individual patient and should be normalised to a body size-related factor as a surrogate for the convective dialysis dose [26], but given that they varied a lot between the studies, research is still needed to set the required cut-off values in the years to come [23].

Acknowledgements

The authors would like to thank Dr. Aileen Grassmann, Director Clinical and Epidemiological Research, Fresenius Medical Care Deutschland GmbH for having the chapter critically reviewed; Prof. Bernard Canaud and Dipl. Ing. Angelica Kneppel for providing the figures; and Sanja Kozlik, NephroCare Manager, Bosnia and Herzegovina for covering the publication fee.

Author details

Goran Imamović[1,2*], Bernard Canaud[3,4], Nusret Mehmedović[5] and Cäcilia Scholz[6]

*Address all correspondence to: goran.imamovic@fmc-ag.com

1 Fresenius Medical Care, Deutschland GmbH, Germany

2 School of Medicine, University of Tuzla, Tuzla, Bosnia and Herzegovina

3 Centre of Excellence Medical, FMC-EMEA, Bad Homburg, Germany

4 School of Medicine, Montpellier University, Montpellier, France

5 Fresenius Medical Care, Bosnia and Herzegovina GmbH, Bosnia and Herzegovina

6 Fresenius Medical Care, Deutschland GmbH, Germany

References

[1] Yavuz, A., et al., Uremic toxins: a new focus on an old subject. Semin Dial, 2005. 18(3): p. 203-11.

[2] Lowrie, E.G., et al., Effect of the hemodialysis prescription of patient morbidity: report from the National Cooperative Dialysis Study. N Engl J Med, 1981. 305(20): p. 1176–81.

[3] The United Renal Data System, Overall hospitalization and mortality. Am J Kidney Dis, 2010. 55(Suppl 1): p. S1.

[4] Collins, A.J., et al., Excerpts from the US Renal Data System 2009 Annual Data Report. Am J Kidney Dis, 2010. 55(1 Suppl 1): p. S1–420, a6–7.

[5] Lowrie, E.G., N.M. Laird, and R.R. Henry, Protocol for the National Cooperative Dialysis Study. Kidney Int Suppl, 1983(13): p. S11-8.

[6] Eknoyan, G., et al., Effect of dialysis dose and membrane flux in maintenance hemodialysis. N Engl J Med, 2002. 347(25): p. 2010–9.

[7] Winchester, J.F., J.A. Salsberg, and N.W. Levin, Beta-2 microglobulin in ESRD: an in-depth review. Adv Ren Replace Ther, 2003. 10(4): p. 279–309.

[8] K/DOQI clinical practice guidelines for bone metabolism and disease in chronic kidney disease . Am J Kidney Dis, 2003. 42(4 Suppl 3): p. S1-201.

[9] Gejyo, F., et al., Beta 2-microglobulin: a new form of amyloid protein associated with chronic hemodialysis. Kidney Int, 1986. 30(3): p. 385–390.

[10] Koch, K.M., Dialysis-related amyloidosis. Kidney Int, 1992. 41(5): p. 1416–29.

[11] Miyata, T., et al., Beta-2 microglobulin in renal disease. J Am Soc Nephrol, 1998. 9(9): p. 1723–35.

[12] Locatelli, F., et al., Effect of membrane permeability on survival of hemodialysis patients. J Am Soc Nephrol, 2009. 20(3): p. 645–54.

[13] Canaud, B., et al., Evaluation of high-flux hemodiafiltration efficiency using an on-line urea monitor. Am J Kidney Dis, 1998. 31(1): p. 74–80.

[14] Canaud, B., et al., Mortality risk for patients receiving hemodiafiltration versus hemodialysis: European results from the DOPPS. Kidney Int, 2006. 69(11): p. 2087–93.

[15] Santoro, A., Mancini, E., MAMHEBI Study Group. Effects of online hemofiltration (OL-HF) versus bicarbonate dialysis (BD) on mortality and morbidity in hemodialysis (HD) patients: a prospective, randomized, multicenter trial (MAMHEBI study). J Am Soc Nephrol, 2006. 17: p. 24

[16] Vilar, E., et al., Long-term outcomes in online hemodiafiltration and high-flux hemodialysis: a comparative analysis. Clin J Am Soc Nephrol, 2009. 4(12): p. 1944–53.

[17] Imamović, G., et al., Survival of incident patients on high-volume online hemodiafiltration compared to low-volume online hemodiafiltration and high-flux hemodialysis. Int Urol Nephrol, 2014. 46(6): p. 1191–200.

[18] Stenvinkel, P., Inflammation in end-stage renal disease – a fire that burns within. Contrib Nephrol, 2005. 149: p. 185–99.

[19] Kjellstrand, C., Kjellstrand, P., Beyond ultrapure hemodialysis: a necessary and achievable goal. Hemodial Int, 2007. 11 (Suppl 1): p. S39.

[20] Ledebo, I., On-line hemodiafiltration: technique and therapy. Adv Ren Replace Ther, 1999. 6(2): p. 195–208.

[21] Ledebo, I., On-line preparation of solutions for dialysis: practical aspects versus safety and regulations. J Am Soc Nephrol, 2002. 13 Suppl 1: p. S78–83.

[22] Vaslaki, L., et al., Can sterile and pyrogen-free on-line substitution fluid be routinely delivered? A multicentric study on the microbiological safety of on-line haemodiafiltration. Nephrol Dial Transplant, 2000. 15 Suppl 1: p. 74–8.

[23] Mostovaya, I.M., et al., Clinical evidence on hemodiafiltration: a systematic review and a meta-analysis. Semin Dial, 2014. 27(2): p. 119–27.

[24] Wizemann, V., et al., Efficacy of haemodiafiltration. Nephrol Dial Transplant, 2001. 16 Suppl 4: p. 27–30.

[25] Maduell, F., et al., Osteocalcin and myoglobin removal in on-line hemodiafiltration versus low- and high-flux hemodialysis. Am J Kidney Dis, 2002. 40(3): p. 582–9.

[26] Tattersall, J.E. and R.A. Ward, Online haemodiafiltration: definition, dose quantification and safety revisited. Nephrol Dial Transplant, 2013. 28(3): p. 542–50.

[27] Lornoy, W., et al., On-line haemodiafiltration. Remarkable removal of beta2-microglobulin. Long-term clinical observations. Nephrol Dial Transplant, 2000. 15 (Suppl 1): p. 49–54.

[28] Lornoy, W., et al., Remarkable removal of beta-2-microglobulin by on-line hemodiafiltration. Am J Nephrol, 1998. 18(2): p. 105–8.

[29] Penne, E.L., et al., Short-term effects of online hemodiafiltration on phosphate control: a result from the randomized controlled Convective Transport Study (CONTRAST). Am J Kidney Dis, 2010. 55(1): p. 77–87.

[30] Beerenhout, C.H., et al., Pre-dilution on-line haemofiltration vs low-flux haemodialysis: a randomized prospective study. Nephrol Dial Transplant, 2005. 20(6): p. 1155–63.

[31] Gatti, E. and C. Ronco, Seeking an optimal renal replacement therapy for the chronic kidney disease epidemic: the case for on-line hemodiafiltration. Contrib Nephrol, 2011. 175: p. 170–85.

[32] Canaud B., K. Pascal, R. Spickermann, and E. Gatti, Online Hemodiafiltration by Fresenius Medical Care. In: Nubé M.J. , Grooteman M.P.C., Blankestijn P., editors. Hemodiafiltration: Theory, Technology and Clinical Practice. 1st ed. Springer International Publishing Switzerland, 2016. p. 95–102.

[33] Potier, J., G. Queffeulou, J. Bouet, Autosub Plus. A sophisticated innovative tool for a simplified OL-HDF practice. Nephrol Dial Transplant Rev (Orlando), 2013. 28 (suppl 1): p. i207.

[34] Donauer, J., et al., Reduction of hypotensive side effects during online-haemodiafiltration and low temperature haemodialysis. Nephrol Dial Transplant, 2003. 18(8): p. 1616–22.

[35] Locatelli, F., et al., Hemofiltration and hemodiafiltration reduce intradialytic hypotension in ESRD. J Am Soc Nephrol, 2010. 21(10): p. 1798–807.

[36] Cheung, A.K., et al., Serum beta-2 microglobulin levels predict mortality in dialysis patients: results of the HEMO study. J Am Soc Nephrol, 2006. 17(2): p. 546–55.

[37] Pedrini, L.A., et al., Long-term effects of high-efficiency on-line haemodiafiltration on uraemic toxicity. A multicentre prospective randomized study. Nephrol Dial Transplant, 2011. 26(8): p. 2617–24.

[38] Di Filippo, S., et al., Sodium removal during pre-dilution haemofiltration. Nephrol Dial Transplant, 2003. 18 Suppl 7: p. vii31–6; discussion vii57–8.

[39] Kawanishi, H., A.C. Yamashita, Haemodiafiltration: A New Era. Karger, 2011.

[40] Zehnder, C., et al., Influence of long-term amelioration of anemia and blood pressure control on left ventricular hypertrophy in hemodialyzed patients. Nephron, 1992. 61(1): p. 21–5.

[41] Ok, E., et al., Mortality and cardiovascular events in online haemodiafiltration (OL-HDF) compared with high-flux dialysis: results from the Turkish OL-HDF Study. Nephrol Dial Transplant, 2013. 28(1): p. 192–202.

[42] Penne, E.L., et al., Effect of increased convective clearance by on-line hemodiafiltration on all cause and cardiovascular mortality in chronic hemodialysis patients - the Dutch CONvective TRAnsport STudy (CONTRAST): rationale and design of a randomised controlled trial [ISRCTN38365125]. Curr Control Trials Cardiovasc Med, 2005. 6(1): p. 8.

[43] Maduell, F., et al., High-efficiency postdilution online hemodiafiltration reduces all-cause mortality in hemodialysis patients. J Am Soc Nephrol, 2013. 24(3): p. 487–97.

[44] Canaud, B., et al., Optimal convection volume for improving patient outcomes in an international incident dialysis cohort treated with online hemodiafiltration. Kidney Int, 2015. 88(5): p. 1108–16.

Chapter 3

Fluid Convection, Generation and Reinfusion in Haemodiafiltration

Emily J. See, Carmel M. Hawley, John WM. Agar and David W. Johnson

Additional information is available at the end of the chapter

http://dx.doi.org/10.5772/62886

Abstract

Despite widespread use in clinical practice for over 30 years, many questions remain unanswered regarding fluid convection and reinfusion strategies in haemodiafiltration (HDF). Randomised controlled trials have failed to consistently demonstrate improved survival with convective therapies, but a dose-dependent improvement in outcome has been suggested. The 'minimum' and 'ideal' volumes of convection are undefined. Online generation of ultrapure dialysis fluid has allowed unprecedented convection volumes; however, delivery of fluid directly into the blood circuit requires strict monitoring. The replacement fluid may be reinfused at multiple points in the circuit. Post-dilution HDF is highly efficient in terms of solute clearance but is limited by haemoconcentration. Pre-dilution HDF prolongs filter life but requires significant convection volumes to achieve adequate solute clearance. Mid-dilution HDF utilises a specific dialyser, which is associated with additional cost and escalating transmembrane pressure. Mixed-dilution HDF appears to offer an attractive balance between solute clearance efficiency and haemoconcentration, however these findings need to be confirmed in large studies. The majority of trials comparing fluid reinfusion strategies have enrolled small numbers of patients over brief study periods. It is unclear whether high-quality evidence examining fluid convection and reinfusion will become available and practice may need to rely on observational data.

Keywords: convection, online fluid generation, reinfusion, haemodiafiltration, end-stage renal disease, outcomes, adverse effects, haemodiafiltration methods, haemodialysis solutions

1. Introduction

With its innovative integration of convective and diffusive techniques, haemodiafiltration (HDF) enhances solute removal across a broad molecular-weight spectrum, which theoretically may improve patient outcomes. Solute clearance by convection requires substantial volumes of ultrafiltration, which in turn necessitates the administration of exogenous fluid replacement. Whilst this fluid may originate from multiple sources, current practice centres around the online generation of sterile, ultrapure dialysate which may be reinfused directly into the circulation. This process requires strict water quality and safety monitoring but enables reinfusion of unlimited volumes of substitution fluid, traditionally either before (pre-dilution HDF) or after (post-dilution HDF) the dialyser. In recent years, two novel HDF techniques (mixed- and mid-dilution HDF) have been developed which permit simultaneous pre- and post-dilution. Both the optimal 'dose' of convection and the ideal site of fluid reinfusion are yet to be determined. This chapter will discuss the evidence surrounding these topics in contemporary HDF practice.

2. Fluid convection

Convective solute transport occurs due to the sieving of solutes across an open membrane in the context of large volumes of ultrafiltration. To achieve maximal convective flux, the volume of ultrafiltration must be optimised. The total volume of ultrafiltration is determined by the ultrafiltration rate and treatment time and is referred to as the convection volume. This value is related to, but distinct from, the substitution volume, which is the quantity of replacement fluid reinfused into the circuit. The difference between the two represents the net fluid removal during the treatment.

Significant changes in the magnitude of the convection volume have taken place since the inception of HDF in the 1970s. Classic HDF used an average substitution volume of 9 L per session, which was primarily limited by cost and logistical issues associated with commercially produced replacement fluid. This is comparable to the estimated amount of convection that occurs during high-flux haemodialysis (HD) today. Most recently, innovations in fluid generation have allowed online production of substitution fluid, which has facilitated convection volumes of 25–40 L per session (and up to 60 L, depending on the mode). This advance has revolutionised the practice of HDF and has piqued interest in the modality worldwide. Importantly, parallel advances in fluid balancing systems have permitted the safe and accurate regulation of ultrafiltration, even at these exceptionally high volumes.

Recently, EUDIAL has set a minimum convection volume for a treatment to be classified as HDF. This threshold is equivalent to 20% of the total processed blood volume [1]. For example, a 4-h treatment with a blood flow rate of 350 ml/min (~84 L/treatment) must have a minimum convection volume of 17 L. Below this, the treatment would be classified as high-flux HD. In general, the convection volume in the post-dilution HDF should be between 17 and 27 L per session [2].

http://dx.doi.org/10.5772/62886

Due to the obvious impact on solute clearance efficiency, the convection volume must be standardised according to the site of fluid reinfusion. This corrected value is termed the *effective convection volume*. In post-dilution HDF, the effective convection volume is the same as the ultrafiltration volume. In mid-dilution HDF, conversion reference tables are provided by the manufacturer. In pre- and mixed-dilution HDF, the ultrafiltration volume must be standardised using a dilution factor (DF) [1]. This is calculated using the plasma water flow rate (Q_{pw}), upstream reinfusion flow rate (Q_{inf}), blood flow rate (Q_b), haematocrit (Hct) and protocrit (Pct) according to the equation:

$$DF = \frac{Q_{pw}}{Q_{pw} + Q_{inf}}$$

$$Q_{pw} = Q_b \times (1 - Hct) \times (1 - 0.016 - Pct)$$

$$N.B.(1 - 0.016 - Pct)\,is\ approximated\ to\ 0.93.$$

2.1. Determinants of convection volume

The maximal achieved convection volume is dependent on several patient- and treatment-related factors, the most important of which are treatment time and blood flow rate (**Table 1**). Other determinants include the transmembrane pressure gradient (TMP), specific characteristics of the dialyser (e.g. membrane surface area, UF coefficient, capillary dimensions, biocompatibility), haematocrit and serum albumin [3, 4]. The term *filtration fraction* is used to describe the ratio between the ultrafiltration rate and the blood flow rate. In post-dilution HDF, it is limited to <0.3 to avoid complications relating to haemoconcentration, namely membrane clotting and high TMP.

Increase convection volume	High blood flow rate
	Long treatment time
	High filtration fraction
	Large membrane surface area
	Biocompatible dialyser
	High UF co-efficient
Decrease convection volume	Hypoalbuminaemia
	Poor vascular access
	High haematocrit
	Small calibre membrane fibres

Table 1. Determinants of convection volume.

2.2. Effect of convection volume on patient outcome

Whilst an overall survival benefit favouring convective therapies has not been established, several studies have supported a 'dose–response' relationship between convection volume and survival (**Table 2**). The Dialysis Outcomes and Practice Patterns Study (DOPPS) first suggested this effect when it showed a 35% relative risk (RR) reduction in mortality between HDF with substitution volumes of 15–25 L and low-flux HD [5]. Since then, there have been three large randomised controlled trials published with similar findings—the CONvective TRAnsport STudy (CONTRAST) [6], the Turkish HDF study [4] and the Estudio de Supervivencia de Hemodiafiltración On-Line (ESHOL) study [7]. In the post hoc analyses of the CONTRAST and the Turkish HDF study, patients with the highest convection volumes were shown to have a survival benefit [4, 8]. In CONTRAST, this difference was seen in the tertile of patients treated with convection volumes >21.95 L (hazard ratio (HR) 0.61) and in the Turkish HDF study, it was seen in patients with a substitution volume >17.4 L (HR 0.54). The ESHOL study demonstrated a similar dose–response effect in its primary analysis: patients treated with convection volumes above 23.1 L had improved all-cause and cardiovascular mortality (HR 0.60) with a further improvement seen at convection volumes >25.4L (HR 0.55) [7]. Further supporting a dose-dependent effect, a pooled analysis of CONTRAST, the Turkish HDF study, the ESHOL study and a French HDF study demonstrated a statistically significant reduction in all-cause mortality in patients receiving the highest convection volumes (24.4–27.4 L) compared with standard HD [8].

The effect of cumulative convection dose on survival has recently been investigated by a retrospective observational study of incident HDF patients. They showed an association between weekly convection volume and survival which began to be apparent at 55 L/week (30 L/week/m^2) and plateaued at 70–75 L/week (40–45 L/week/m^2) [9]. This is the first paper to recognise the importance of cumulative treatment dose, taking into account session frequency, which may be particularly relevant to mortality outcomes.

	Substitution volume	**Convection volume**	**RR or HR (CI)**
DOPPS [5]	>15 L/session	>17.5 L/session	0.65
CONTRAST [6]	>19.45 L/session	>21.95 L/session	0.61 (0.38–0.98)
TURKISH OL-HDF [4]	>17.4 L/session	>19.9 L/session	0.54 (0.31–0.93)
ESHOL [7]	20.6–22.9 L/session	23.1–25.4 L/session	0.60 (0.39–0.90)
	>22.9 L/session	>25.4 L/session	0.55 (0.34–0.84)

Table 2. Volumes required to achieve a reduction in mortality (expressed as RR or HR with confidence interval (CI), and assuming an average net fluid removal of 2.5 L).

2.3. Assessment of adequate solute clearance

Assessment of HDF adequacy must take into account removal of solutes across all molecular weights. Specifically, enhanced middle- and large-molecule clearance should not occur at the expense of inferior small-solute clearance. For practical purposes, small-solute clearance should be quantified using the same approach as for HD, whether that be calculation of Kt/V_{urea} or percentage reduction in urea. Of note, blood samples must be taken upstream of any fluid reinfusion port to avoid sample dilution. This is especially relevant in the pre-dilution and mixed-dilution HDF modes where substitution fluid is infused before the dialyser. In terms of assessing middle-molecule clearance, convective dialysis 'dose' appears to be a linear function of substitution volume so reporting of this value is routinely used [11, 12].

2.4. Consequences of high convection volume

Due to the indiscriminate nature of solute removal by large-volume ultrafiltration, inadvertent removal of beneficial solutes is unavoidable. The most significant example of this is albumin. The degree of albumin loss in a HDF treatment is dependent on the membrane type, ultrafiltration volume and TMP. The site of fluid reinfusion is also relevant as a key determinant of ultrafiltration volume and TMP; the use of post- and mid-dilution HDF may increase the loss of albumin up to fivefold [12]. Albumin removal can be minimised by profiled filtration modes, which limit initial filtration, or by regulated TMP control. Fortunately, as described in the randomised trials and observational studies, albumin loss did not appear to affect nutritional parameters or serum albumin concentration [4, 6, 9, 10, 13]. It should therefore not limit the utilisation of HDF or the prescribed convection volume in current practice, but will require ongoing evaluation in future trials given the lack of robust safety data.

2.5. Individualising convection volume

The requisite 'dose' of convection likely varies between individuals. This in turn has theoretical implications for future trial design and practical implications for HDF prescription. Two important patient characteristics that should be considered are patient size and residual renal function [1]. Having an absolute convection volume target for all patients is not logical since patients vary widely in size, body composition and metabolic rate. Recently, the HDF Pooling Project Investigators looked at the effect of convection volume on mortality when stratified convection volumes were standardised according to patient size. The survival advantage for higher convective dose was maintained after standardising for total body water and body surface areas, which are surrogate markers of lean body mass, but not for body weight or body mass index [8]. Other patient factors may also be important in determining optimal convection volume including age, ethnic background, comorbidity index, diabetic status and dialysis vintage. The importance of these additional factors is yet to be studied.

3. Substitution fluid

The degree of ultrafiltration that occurs in HDF necessitates reinfusion of large volumes of replacement fluid into the extracorporeal circuit. This fluid must be sterile and non-pyrogenic with a biochemical composition similar to plasma water. The replacement fluid may be obtained in two ways: internal substitution (e.g. internal filtration HDF, push–pull HDF, double high-flux HDF and paired filtration dialysis) or external substitution (e.g. classic HDF and online HDF).

3.1. Internal substitution

3.1.1. Internal filtration HDF

Internal filtration HDF uses pressure profiling to take advantage of the substantial volumes of plasma water that can be filtered across high-flux dialysers. Difference in pressure between the blood and dialysate compartments results in proximal ultrafiltration followed by distal backfiltration (**Figure 1**). Backfiltration of dialysate is analogous to reinfusion of substitution fluid. Sudden shifts in plasma water may lead to increased rates of haemolysis. Backfiltration poses an additional risk of biological and endotoxin contamination; however, the use of dialysis membranes with a high endotoxin retention capacity minimises this risk.

3.1.2. Push–pull HDF

Push–pull HDF involves rapid alternations in ultrafiltration and backfiltration across a single high-flux dialyser using a double-pump system installed on the effluent line (**Figure 1**). These alternations are controlled by fluctuations in pressure that occur due to varying the volume of the dialysate compartment. Fluid is reinfused along the course of the dialyser, favouring the blood outlet port where the pressure in the blood compartment is lowest. The convection volume may be as high as 120 L throughout a standard 4 h treatment [14]. Albumin loss is significantly lower than In post-dilution HDF due to lower TMP [15]. Intermittent backfiltra-

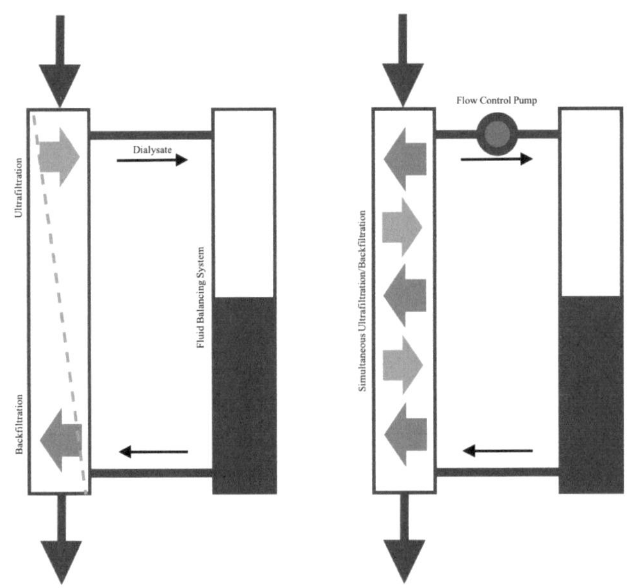

Figure 1. Internal filtration HDF and push-pull HDF.

tion removes protein deposition on the blood side of the membrane making this technique also suitable for extended-hour renal replacement therapy (e.g. nocturnal or continuous HDF).

3.1.3. *Double high-flux HDF*

Double high-flux HDF consists of two high-flux membranes connected in series and subjected to high blood and dialysate flow rates (**Figure 2**). Simultaneous diffusion and convection occur across the first membrane, whilst backfiltration of sterile dialysate occurs across the second. Variation in pressure and flow across the two dialysers is controlled by a resistance valve. Using this system, von Albertini was able to achieve 13 L convection per 2 h treatment and significant clearances of both small and larger solutes [16].

3.1.4. *Paired filtration dialysis*

Paired filtration dialysis uses two high-flux membranes connected in series. The first is a haemofilter with a small surface area, which performs ultrafiltration, and the second is a haemodialyser which performs diffusion. The substitution fluid is infused between the two. The main variation of this technique is paired filtration dialysis with endogenous reinfusion. This is also referred to as haemodiafiltration with endogenous reinfusion (HFR): In HFR, ultrafiltrate passes through a purifying charcoal/resin filter before being reinfused as substitution fluid (**Figure 2**).

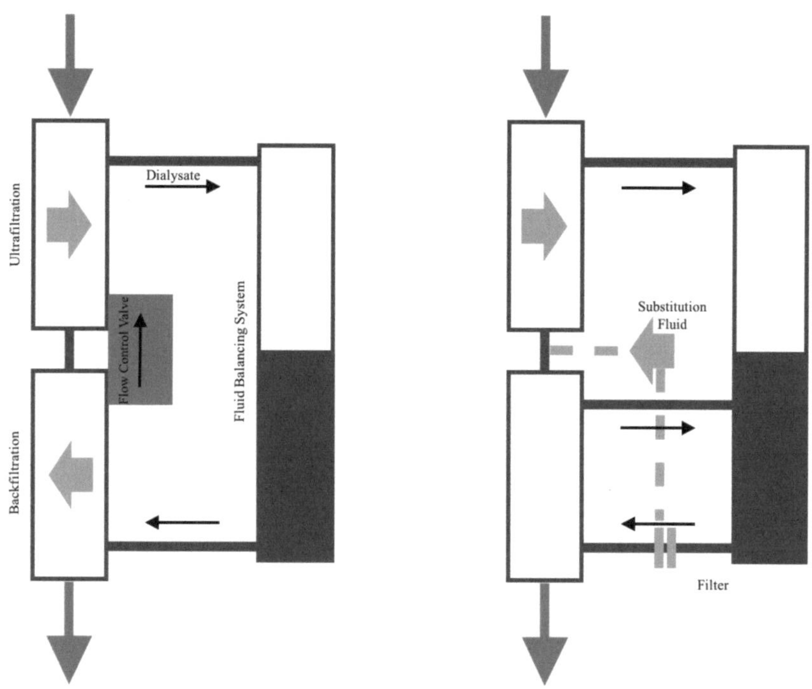

Figure 2. Double high-flux HDF and paired filtration dialysis with endogenous reinfusion.

3.1.5. Classic HDF

Classic HDF consists of a single dialyser which performs haemodiafiltration. The convection volume is replaced with packaged, commercially produced substitution fluid which is reinfused after the dialyser (**Figure 3**). This practice is associated with significant expense and obvious logistic issues [17]. These factors limit the volume of convection and therefore solute clearance.

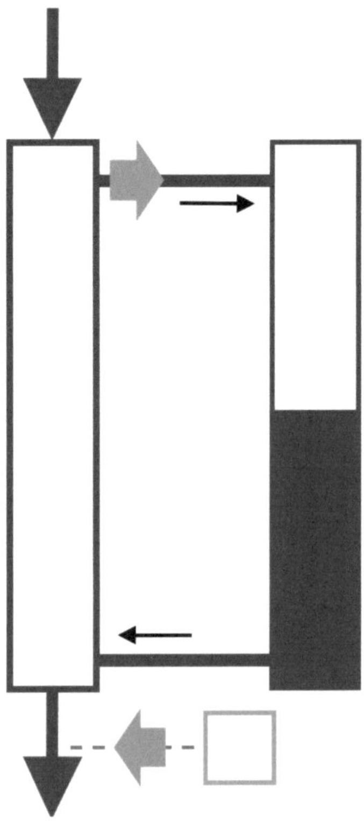

Figure 3. Classic HDF.

3.1.6. Online HDF

Online HDF relies on the ability of modern dialysis machines to generate unlimited quantities of ultrapure dialysis fluid, which can be reinfused directly into the circulation. In this system, dialysis fluid is prepared by the proportioning of ultrapure water and a concentrated electrolyte solution. This fluid is then used as both dialysate and substitution fluid (**Figures 6** and **7**). The integrity of the chemical composition is monitored using conductivity measurements. First described in the 1970s, the development of online fluid generation has facilitated the evolution of HDF from low-volume to high-volume practice [18]. It has been commercially available for over a decade and comes at minimal additional cost compared to high flux HD. This modality is the most widely utilised HDF technique in contemporary dialysis. It is well established in

Europe and Japan, and is experiencing escalating use in Australia and New Zealand (currently representing 16% of haemodialysis modalities) [19].

3.2. Biological safety

Since significant quantities of substitution fluid are being reinfused directly into the blood circuit, strict biological safety is essential. Many countries have specific policies outlining the technical requirements and water monitoring processes that dialysis units must comply with to practice HDF. Additionally, international guidelines exist which underpin the minimum standards for microbiological and chemical quality [20]. These technical requirements include the use of specific HDF machines and the ability to generate ultrapure water and dialysis fluid (**Table 3**). Generation of ultrapure water involves a pre-treatment system (microfiltration, softeners, activated carbon) followed by two reverse osmosis modules connected in series (**Figure 4**). In some water treatment systems, the reverse osmosis modules will be followed by a storage tank.

	Regular water	Ultrapure water	Ultrapure dialysate
Microbial contamination	<100 CFU/ml	<0.1 CFU/ml	<0.1 CFU/ml
Bacterial endotoxins	<0.25 IU/ml	<0.03 IU/ml	<0.03 IU/ml

Table 3. Water purity definitions.

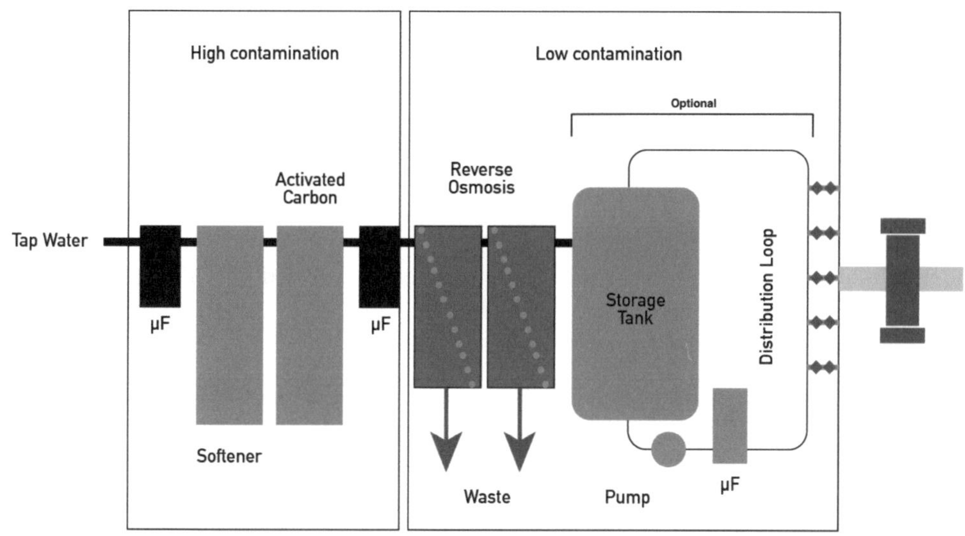

Figure 4. Conversion of tap water to ultrapure water.

Ultrapure water is converted to ultrapure dialysis fluid by combination with an electrolyte concentrate. The fluid then undergoes cold sterilisation, a process involving a series of filters with bacterial and endotoxin retentive properties at intermediate points in the circuit. An inbuilt infusion pump diverts a proportion of ultrapure dialysate through another safety filter prior to being directly infused into the patient's bloodstream as replacement fluid (**Figure 5**).

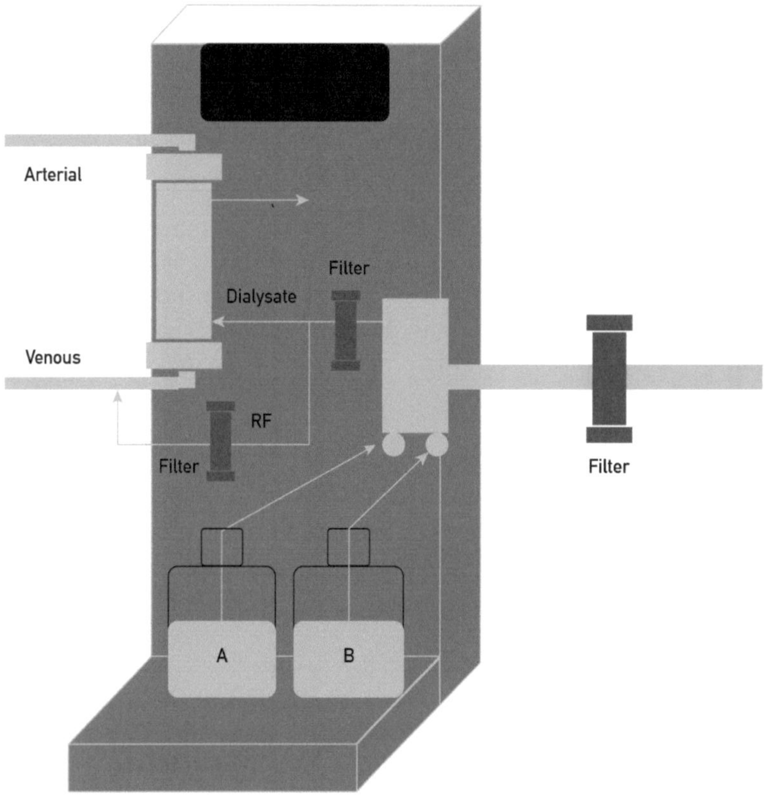

Figure 5. Conversion of ultrapure water to ultrapure dialysate.

Beyond the actual production of ultrapure dialysate, frequent disinfection of the water treatment system and dialysis machine, Thermochemical destruction of the biofilm, regular change of filters and maintenance of a permanent circulation of water are essential. Microbiological and endotoxin monitoring must also be carried out.

Several clinical studies have confirmed the safety of online HDF provided that appropriate CE marked and certified HDF machines are used and the best clinical practices are applied [21]. The three largest RCTs comparing HDF to HD did not demonstrate any higher incidence of infectious complications using online fluid generation [4, 8, 9].

4. Site of fluid reinfusion

Online HDF modalities are classified according to the location at which the replacement fluid is administered in the extracorporeal circuit. The replacement fluid has traditionally been reinfused either before (pre-dilution) or after (post-dilution) the dialyser. Simultaneous pre- and post-dilution HDF techniques (mixed- and mid-dilution) have gained popularity in recent years. Each has relative advantages and disadvantages (**Table 4**). Other novel hybrid modalities have been proposed including 'pre-dilution on demand' and 'backflush on demand'.

	Post-dilution	Pre-dilution	Mixed-dilution	Mid-dilution
Small-solute clearance	+++	+	+++	++
Medium solute clearance	++	+	+++	+++
Protein-bound solute clearance	++	+	+++	++
Albumin loss	++	+	+	+++
Filter clotting	++	+	+	+++
High TMP	++	+	+	+++

Table 4. Relative advantages and disadvantages of fluid reinfusion site.

4.1. Post-dilution HDF

Post-dilution HDF is regarded as the most efficient form of HDF in terms of solute clearance and is the most common format used in contemporary clinical practice. By reinfusing fluid after the dialyser, a continuous concentration gradient is maintained along the entire course of the dialyser (**Figure 6**). This approach has been shown to be superior to both high-flux HD and pre-dilution HDF in terms of small-solute and middle-molecule clearance [11, 22].

The efficiency of solute clearance in this system occurs at the expense of escalating haemoconcentration, which increases the risk of filter clotting, membrane pore occlusion and a subsequent increase in TMP. In extreme cases, red cell damage and protein denaturation may occur. There is also an increased risk of albumin loss as a result of the high TMP. The potential for haemoconcentration means that the filtration fraction must be limited which in turn necessitates a high blood flow rate to achieve adequate convection (typically >350 ml/min). Therefore, in patients with poor vascular access, inadequate blood flow may compromise the ability to achieve satisfactory clearances. Similarly, the risk of filter clotting means that patients with high haematocrit, cryoglobulinemia or gammopathy should be preferentially managed with pre-dilution or mixed-dilution HDF.

4.2. Pre-dilution HDF

In pre-dilution HDF, the substitution fluid is reinfused before the entry of blood into the dialyser (**Figure 6**). This avoids complications relating to haemoconcentration which extends filter life and lowers TMP. Because of the lower risk of clotting, heparin dose can be minimised and heparin-free dialysis for high-risk patients is possible [23]. In Japan, where this technique is used most widely, improvements in shear stress, blood pressure and haematological parameters (especially neutrophil and lymphocyte function) have also been reported [24, 25].

This same group have described improvements in dialysis-related symptom burden including itch, restless legs syndrome and insomnia compared to the post-dilution HDF.

Pre-dilution HDF has obvious deleterious effects on the efficiency of solute clearance. The reduced efficiency of this system means that ultrafiltration rates must be at least twofold higher than those in post-dilution HDF to achieve equivalent solute clearance. In fact, ultrafiltration rates of up to 100% of the blood flow rate are often used.

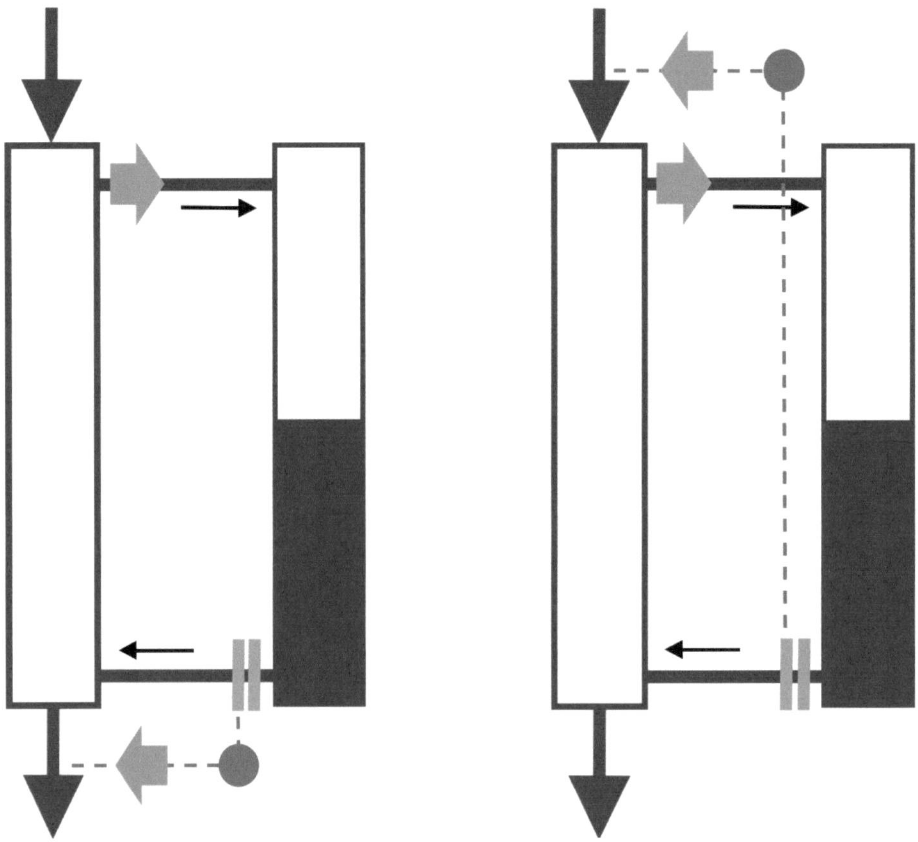

Figure 6. Post-dilution HDF and pre-dilution HDF.

4.3. Mixed-dilution HDF

In mixed-dilution HDF, fluid is simultaneously reinfused both before and after the dialyser in a ratio that is automatically regulated by the TMP and ultrafiltration feedback (**Figure 7**). An internal feedback mechanism maintains the TMP between 250 and 300 mmHg and ensures a maximum filtration fraction after considering the blood and dialysate flow, internal pressure and hydraulic permeability of the dialyser. Convection volume tends to be 30–40 L/session. TMP is calculated according to the pressure measured at four points in the system: blood entry into the dialyser entry ($P_{blood\ in}$), blood exit from the dialyser ($P_{blood\ out}$), dialysate entry into the dialyser ($P_{dialysate\ in}$) and dialysate exit into the dialyser ($P_{dialysate\ out}$).

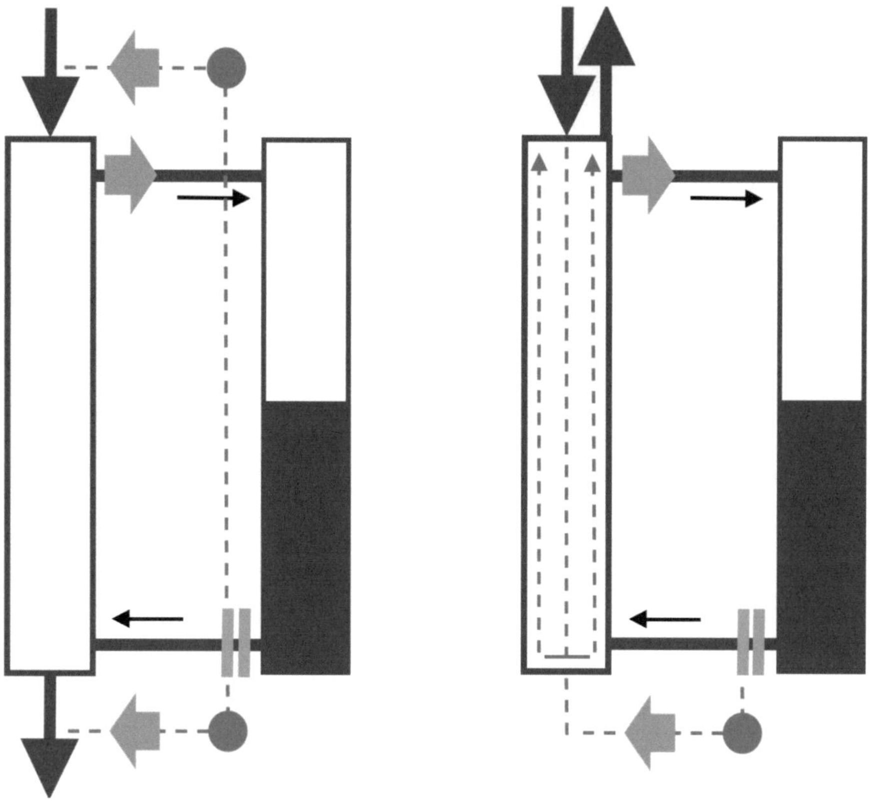

Figure 7. Representation of the mixed-dilution and mid-dilution HDF.

$$TMP = 0.5 \times [(P_{blood\ in} + P_{blood\ out}) - (P_{dialysate\ in} + P_{dialysate\ out})]$$

If the TMP rises beyond its maximum tolerated value, a fraction of infused dialysate is diverted from post- to pre-dilution, which decreases haemoconcentration and lowers the risk of membrane pore occlusion. Similarly, if the TMP falls below the target range, fluid is redirected towards the post-dilution mode to increase system efficiency.

Mixed dilution HDF has been shown to be non-inferior to post-dilution HDF in terms of small and protein-bound solute clearance and superior to post-dilution and pre-dilution HDF in terms of β_2-microglobulin clearance (β_2-M) [26–29]. Whilst these were relatively small randomised trials which require larger studies to confirm their findings, mixed-dilution HDF appears to offer an attractive balance between efficiency of solute removal and minimisation of haemoconcentration-related complications. Specifically, it may be suitable for patients in whom target convection volumes are not achieved by post-dilution HDF because of high haematocrit, high plasma protein, or inadequate vascular access and blood flow rate.

4.4. Mid-dilution HDF

Mid-dilution HDF similarly combines pre- and post-dilution fluid reinfusion into a hybrid system (**Figure 7**). It does so by utilising a specialised haemodiafilter, the Nephros OLpur MD 190. This filter is constructed in such a way that blood enters through the central core fibres of the dialyser and returns in the opposite direction peripherally. This model effectively comprises two dialysers in series. Substitution fluid is incorporated at the midpoint of the system, which creates an initial post-dilution stage followed by a pre-dilution stage. This enables a high-concentration gradient and encourages movement of small solutes in the first stage and maximal ultrafiltration of plasma water and convective removal of larger molecules in the second stage. Reinfusion rates up to 10–12 L/h are possible.

Unfortunately, due to the nature of the specialised dialyser, mid-dilution HDF is associated with higher costs. There is also a higher degree of albumin loss, which is not insignificant. Concerns exist regarding generation of a high TMP, which could compromise membrane permeability. A TMP of up to 1000 mmHg has been reported as necessary to achieve the required minimum ultrafiltration of 6 L/h [30]. This high TMP is especially problematic in the first section of the dialyser where the post-dilution phase takes place and is thought to be the result of partial fibre clotting and increased resistance to blood flow due to the reduced capillary diameter in this segment [31]. Given the pro-coagulant effect of rapid convection, adequate anticoagulation is necessary to ensure device patency. Reversal of the configuration of the blood tubing (i.e. connecting the arterial line to the venous port of the dialyser and vice versa) has been successfully trialled in mid-dilution HDF without significant effect on plasma clearances if adequate infusion rates are maintained [32, 33]. Consideration should also be given to the use of larger-surface filters (e.g. Nephros OLpur MD 220) [34].

When compared to post-dilution HDF, mid-dilution HDF is associated with inferior small solute but superior middle-molecule clearance (β_2M, myoglobin, prolactin, RTP) and similar clearance of protein-bound solutes [35–37]. With increasing molecular weight, differences in treatment efficiency between mid- and post-dilution HDF rise [36]. Phosphate clearance is similar between the two groups. Whilst few studies have compared mid- and mixed-dilution HDF, one small prospective randomised trial found greater small-solute and middle-molecule clearance with mixed-dilution HDF though differences in dialyser membranes may have confounded their outcomes [30]. Another small prospective crossover study compared 'simple mid-dilution' (using two dialysers in series, rather than the Nephros OLpur MD 190) and mixed-dilution HDF. They similarly found that mixed-dilution HDF provided significantly greater clearances of urea, creatinine and β_2M compared To 'simple mid-dilution' HDF with equivalent phosphate clearances [38]. These outcomes require examination in larger trials.

4.5. Novel systems

Two novel systems, *'pre-dilution on demand'* and *'backflush on demand'*, have recently been proposed as potential alternatives to the standard online HDF modalities [39]. These sys-

http://dx.doi.org/10.5772/62886

tems utilise inbuilt automated software to balance ultrafiltration against haemoconcentration. In pre-dilution on-demand mode, escalating TMP is managed by temporarily pausing ultrafiltration and diverting a proportion of filtered dialysate into the dialyser in pre-dilution mode as a bolus. This produces sudden haemodilution. In backflush on demand, rising TMP results in an automatic cessation of filtration and an infusion of ultrapure dialysate into the dialyser. This creates positive pressure in the dialysate compartment, which backflushes the membrane pores and reduces haemoconcentration. These modes are currently experimental but offer a novel and intuitive solution to some of the inherent technical barriers of the existing HDF modes. Of note, these machines and dialysers would carry additional expense, which would need to be considered.

5. Summary

Many questions remain unanswered in the field of fluid convection, generation and reinfusion in haemodiafiltration. Although convection volume appears to have a dose-dependent relationship with survival, randomised trials have failed to consistently demonstrate improved mortality in their primary analyses. Furthermore, the critical 'dose' required to improve patient outcomes is yet to be determined and may need to be individualised according to patient factors, including patient size and residual renal function. Online generation of ultrapure dialysate has revolutionised the practice of HDF by allowing large convection volumes, although this approach requires strict monitoring in terms of quality and safety. The preferred site of fluid reinfusion is not known and warrants careful consideration of the opposing factors of solute clearance efficiency and the consequences of haemoconcentration. Hybrid modalities appear to present a promising balance between the two. Given the lack of robust clinical trials confirming the benefits of HDF, the increasing uptake of HDF worldwide has largely been driven by industry. Lack of a harm signal, cost neutrality and optimism that patient benefits will arise from large convective volumes have facilitated acceptance amongst the Nephrology community. It is unclear whether high-quality data from randomised trials will be available to guide convection and reinfusion strategies and it is likely that practice will need to rely on the results of observational studies.

Author details

Emily J. See[1], Carmel M. Hawley[1], John WM. Agar[2] and David W. Johnson[1*]

*Address all correspondence to: david.johnson2@health.qld.gov.au

1 University of Queensland at Princess Alexandra Hospital, Brisbane, Australia

2 University Hospital Geelong, Geelong, Australia

References

[1] Tattersall JE, Ward RA. Online haemodiafiltration: Definition, dose quantification and safety revisited. Nephrol Dial Transplant. 2013;28:542–50. doi:10.1093/ndt/gfs530.

[2] Mostovaya IM, Blankestijn PJ, Bots ML, Covic A, Davenport A, Grooteman MPC, et al. Clinical evidence on hemodiafiltration: A systematic review and a meta-analysis. Semin Dial. 2014;27:119–27. doi:10.1111/sdi.12200.

[3] Penne EL, van der Weerd NC, Bots ML, van den Dorpel M, Grooteman MPC, Lévesque R, et al. Patient- and treatment-related determinants of convective volume in post-dilution haemodiafiltration in clinical practice. Nephrol Dial Transplant. 2009;24:3493–9. doi:10.1093/ndt/gfp265.

[4] Ok E, Asci G, Toz H, Ok ES, Kircelli F, Yilmaz M, et al. Mortality and cardiovascular events in online haemodiafiltration (OL-HDF) compared with high-flux dialysis: Results from the Turkish OL-HDF Study. Nephrol Dial Transplant. 2013;28:192–202. doi:10.1093/ndt/gfs407.

[5] Canaud B, Bragg-Gresham JL, Marshall MR, Desmeules S, Gillespie BW, Depner T, et al. Mortality risk for patients receiving hemodiafiltration versus hemodialysis: European results from the DOPPS. Kidney Int. 2006;69:2087–93. doi:10.1038/sj.ki.5000447.

[6] Grooteman MPC, van den Dorpel M., Bots ML, Penne EL, van der Weerd NC, Mazairac H, et al. Effect of online hemodiafiltration on all-cause mortality and cardiovascular outcomes. J Am Soc Nephrol. 2012;23:1087–96. doi:10.1681/ASN.2011121140.

[7] Maduell F, Moreso F, Pons M, Ramos R, Mora-Macià J, Carreras J, et al. High-efficiency postdilution online hemodiafiltration reduces all-cause mortality in hemodialysis patients. J Am Soc Nephrol. 2013;24:487–97. doi:10.1681/ASN.2012080875.

[8] Davenport A, Peters SAE, Bots ML, Canaud B, Grooteman MPC, Asci G, et al. Higher convection volume exchange with online hemodiafiltration is associated with survival advantage for dialysis patients: The effect of adjustment for body size. Kidney Int. 2015;89:193–199. doi:10.1038/ki.2015.264.

[9] Canaud B, Barbieri C, Marcelli D, Bellocchio F, Bowry S, Mari F, et al. Optimal convection volume for improving patient outcomes in an international incident dialysis cohort treated with online hemodiafiltration. Kidney Int. 2015;88:1–9. doi:10.1038/ki.2015.139.

[10] Lornoy W, Becaus I, Billiouw JM, Sierens L, Van Malderen P, D'Haenens P. On-line haemodiafiltration. Remarkable removal of beta2-microglobulin. Long-term clinical observations. Nephrol Dial Transplant. 2000;15 (suppl 1):49–54. doi:10.1093/oxfordjournals.ndt.a027964.

[11] Lornoy W, Becaus I, Billiouw J-M, Sierens L, van Malderen P. Remarkable removal of beta-2-microglobulin by on-line hemodiafiltration. Am J Nephrol. 1998;18:105–108. Am J Nephrol. 1998;18:105–8. doi:10.1159/000013317.

[12] Krieter DH, Canaud B. High permeability of dialysis membranes: What is the limit of albumin loss. Nephrol Dial Transplant. 2003;18:651–4. doi:10.1093/ndt/gfg054.

[13] Fournier A, Birmele B, Francois M, Prat L, Halimi J. Factors associated with albumin loss in post-dilution hemodiafiltration and nutritional consequences. Int J Artif Organs. 2015;38:76–82. doi:10.5301/ijao.5000389.

[14] Miwa M, Shinzato T. Push/pull hemodiafiltration: Technical aspects and clinical effectiveness. Artif Organs. 1999;23:1123–6. doi:10.1046/j.1525-1694.1999.06173.x.

[15] Shinzato T, Miwa M, Nakai S, Takai I, Matsumoto Y, Morita H, et al. Alternate repetition of short fore- and backfiltrations reduces convective albumin loss. Kidney Int. 1996;50:432–5. doi:10.1038/ki.1996.333.

[16] von Albertini B, Miller J, Gardner P, Shinaberger J. High-flux hemodiafiltration: Under six hours/week treatment. Trans Am Soc Artif Intern Organs. 1984;30:227–31. doi: 10.1093/ndtplus/sfp149.

[17] Leber HW, Wizemann V, Goubeaud G, Rawer P, Schutterle G. Hemodiafiltration: A new alternative to hemofiltration and conventional hemodialysis. Artif Organs. 1978;2:150–3. doi:10.1111/j.1525-1594.1978.tb03444.x.

[18] Henderson L, Beans E. Successful production of sterile pyrogen-free electrolyte solution by ultrafiltration. Kidney Int. 1978;14:522–5. doi:10.1038/ki.1978.157.

[19] McDonald S. Australia and New Zealand Dialysis and Transplant Registry Report. Chapter 4: Haemodialysis, Adelaide: 2014, p. 4.12.

[20] International Electrotechnical Commission. Particular requirements for basic safety and essential performance of haemodialysis, haemodiafiltration and haemofiltration equipment. 3rd ed. Geneva, Switzerland: 2008. doi:10.3403/30263013.

[21] Vaslaki L, Karátson A, Vörös P, Major L, Pethö F, Ladányi E, et al. Can sterile and pyrogen-free on-line substitution fluid be routinely delivered? A multicentric study on the microbiological safety of on-line haemodiafiltration. Nephrol Dial Transplant. 2000;15 (suppl 1):74–8. doi:10.1111/j.1744-9987.2009.00674.x.

[22] Meert N, Eloot S, Waterloos MA, Van Landschoot M, Dhondt A, Glorieux G, et al. Effective removal of protein-bound uraemic solutes by different convective strategies: A prospective trial. Nephrol Dial Transplant. 2009;24:562–70. doi:10.1093/ndt/gfn522.

[23] Wamsiedler R, Polaschegg HD, Tattersall JE. Heparin-free dialysis with an on-line hemodiafiltration system. Artif Organs. 1993;17:948–50. doi:10.1111/j.1525-1594.1993.tb00408.x.

[24] Sakurai K, Saito T, Yamauchi F, Asahi D, Hosoya H. Comparison of the effects of predilution and postdilution hemodiafiltration on neutrophils, lymphocytes and platelets. J Artif Organs. 2013;16:316–21. doi:10.1007/s10047-013-0698-0.

[25] Locatelli F, Altieri P, Andrulli S, Bolasco P, Sau G, Pedrini L a, et al. Hemofiltration and hemodiafiltration reduce intradialytic hypotension in ESRD. J Am Soc Nephrol. 2010;21:1798–807. doi:10.1681/ASN.2010030280.

[26] de Sequera P, Albalate M, Pérez-García R, Corchete E, Puerta M, Ortega M, et al. A comparison of the effectiveness of two online haemodiafiltration modalities: Mixed versus post-dilution. Nefrologia. 2013;33:779–87. doi:10.3265/Nefrologia.pre2013.Sep.12223.

[27] Pedrini L, De Cristofaro V, Pagliari B, Samà F. Mixed predilution and postdilution online hemodiafiltration compared with the traditional infusion modes. Kidney Int. 2000;58:2155–65. doi:10.1111/j.1523-1755.2000.00389.x.

[28] Potier J, Le Roy F, Faucon JP, Besselièvre T, Renaudineau E, Farquet C, et al. Elevated removal of middle molecules without significant albumin loss with mixed-dilution hemodiafiltration for patients unable to provide sufficient blood flow rates. Blood Purif. 2013;36:78–83. doi:10.1159/000351527.

[29] Pedrini L, De Cristofaro V. On-line mixed hemodiafiltration with a feedback for ultrafiltration control: Effect on middle-molecule removal. Kidney Int. 2003;64:1505–13. doi:10.1046/j.1523-1755.2003.00240.x.

[30] Feliciani A, Riva MA, Zerbi S, Ruggiero P, Plati AR, Cozzi G, et al. New strategies in haemodiafiltration (HDF): Prospective comparative analysis between on-line mixed HDF and mid-dilution HDF. Nephrol Dial Transplant. 2007;22:1672–9. doi:10.1093/ndt/gfm023.

[31] Feliciani A, Pedrini L. New strategies in haemodiafiltration (HDF): Prospective comparative analysis between on-line mixed HDF and mid-dilution HDF. Nephrol Dial Transplant. 2008;23:1466. doi:10.1093/ndt/gfm841.

[32] Krieter DH, Canaud B. New strategies in haemodialfiltration (HDF)—Prospective comparative analysis between online mixed HDF and mid-dilution HDF. Nephrol Dial Transplant. 2008;23:1465–6. doi:10.1093/ndt/gfm604.

[33] Santoro A, Ferramosca E, Mancini E, Monari C, Varasani M, Sereni L, et al. Reverse mid-dilution: New way to remove small and middle molecules as well as phosphate with high intrafilter convective clearance. Nephrol Dial Transplant. 2007;22:2000–5. doi:10.1093/ndt/gfm101.

[34] Pedrini L, Feliciani A, Zerbi S, Cozzi G, Ruggiero P. Optimization of mid-dilution haemodiafiltration: Technique and performance. Nephrol Dial Transplant. 2009;24:2816–24. doi:10.1093/ndt/gfp207.

[35] Maduell F, Arias M, Vera M, Fontseré N, Blasco M, Barros X, et al. Mid-dilution hemodiafiltration: A comparison with pre- and postdilution modes using the same polyphenylene membrane. Blood Purif. 2009;28:268–74. doi:10.1159/000232935.

[36] Krieter DH, Falkenhain S, Chalabi L, Collins G, Lemke H-D, Canaud B. Clinical cross-over comparison of mid-dilution hemodiafiltration using a novel dialyzer concept and

post-dilution hemodiafiltration. Kidney Int. 2005;67:349–56. doi:10.1111/j.1523-1755.2005.00088.x.

[37] Eloot S, Dhondt A, Van Landschoot M, Waterloos MA, Vanholder R. Removal of water-soluble and protein-bound solutes with reversed mid-dilution versus post-dilution haemodiafiltration. Nephrol Dial Transplant. 2012;27:3278–83. doi:10.1093/ndt/gfs060.

[38] Susantitaphong P, Tiranathanagul K, Katavetin P, Hanwiwatwong O, Wittayalertpanya S, Praditpornsilpa K, et al. Efficacy comparison between simple mixed-dilution and simple mid-dilution on-line hemodiafiltration techniques: A crossover study. Artif Organs. 2012;36:1059–65. doi:10.1111/j.1525-1594.2012.01508.x.

[39] Ronco C, Cruz D. Hemodiafiltration: Technical and clinical issues. Adv Chronic Kidney Dis. 2015;14:231–43. doi:10.1159/000437403.

Chapter 4

The Effect of Convective Dialytic Modalities on Arterial Stiffness in End-Stage Renal Disease Patients

Panagiotis I. Georgianos, Evangelia Dounousi,
Theodoros Eleftheriadis and Vassilios Liakopoulos

Additional information is available at the end of the chapter

http://dx.doi.org/10.5772/63369

Abstract

Among end-stage renal disease (ESRD) patients receiving hemodialysis, increased arterial stiffness is an independent cardiovascular risk predictor. Over the past few years, arterial stiffness attenuation has been increasingly recognized as a novel therapeutic target toward cardiovascular risk reduction in the dialysis population. Structural alterations related to the long-term arteriosclerotic process are difficult to modify; with the exception of blood pressure (BP)-lowering, there are no other therapeutic interventions with well-documented benefits in delaying the progression of arteriosclerosis among dialysis patients. Enhanced clearance of middle-to-high molecular weight solutes by combining convective and diffusive transport through hemodiafiltration and the associated benefits on microvascular endothelial function have generated the hypothesis that convective dialytic modalities may be advantageous in improving large-artery stiffness. This notion is supported by some clinical studies showing that switching ESRD patients from low-flux hemodialysis to high-efficiency on-line hemodiafiltration was associated with significant reduction in arterial stiffness. These beneficial effects, however, were not confirmed in a recent subanalysis of the CONvective TRAnsport STudy (CONTRAST) trial. In this chapter, we summarize the currently available evidence on the effect of hemodiafiltration versus hemodialysis on arterial stiffness, discussing also the potential clinical implications of this effect.

Keywords: arterial stiffness, hemodiafiltration, hemodialysis, pulse wave velocity, vascular calcification

1. Introduction

Patients with end-stage-renal-disease (ESRD) receiving maintenance hemodialysis have one of the highest rates of cardiovascular morbidity and mortality [1, 2]. Although classical atheromatosis of middle-sized arteries is an important contributor to this elevated cardiovascular risk, atherosclerotic cardiovascular events (i.e., myocardial infarction and stroke) can only partially explain the huge burden of cardiovascular mortality in ESRD. Among these patients, serious arrhythmias and sudden cardiac deaths related to the high prevalence of left ventricular (LV) hypertrophy and disturbances in electrolyte balance represent another major cause of cardiovascular death [3]. This phenomenon is explained by the fact that the spectrum of arterial remodeling in ESRD is much broader, including also long-term structural alterations in the visco-elastic properties of the biomaterial constituting the wall of the aorta and large conduit arteries [4, 5]. The so-called "arteriosclerotic process" is accompanied by substantial hemodynamic alterations and is considered one of the most important pathogenic mechanisms of isolated systolic hypertension, LV hypertrophy, and subendocardial hypoperfusion [4, 5]. It is therefore unsurprising that among ESRD patients, increased arterial stiffness is a strong and powerful predictor of cardiovascular morbidity and mortality [6, 7].

Given the strong prognostic association of arterial stiffness with cardiovascular outcomes, regression of the arteriosclerotic process is increasingly recognized as a novel therapeutic target toward cardiovascular risk reduction in dialysis patients. However, whether arterial stiffness in this particular population is modifiable and if so, which therapeutic interventions are effective in delaying the progression of arteriosclerosis are aspects that remain unclear [5, 8]. Observational evidence and a few randomized studies suggested that blood pressure (BP)-lowering and use of agents blocking the renin-angiotensin-aldosterone-system (RAAS) may be of some benefit [5, 8, 9]. The modality of renal replacement therapy is suggested to be another factor possibly determining the progression of arteriosclerosis in dialysis patients. In this regard, higher clearance of middle-to-large molecular weight solutes by combining diffusive and convective transport and the associated improvement in phosphate control, endothelial dysfunction, and circulating inflammatory biomarkers [10–14] is proposed to be translated into a beneficial impact of hemodiafiltration on large-artery structure and function in dialysis patients.

The aim of this chapter was to review the currently available evidence on the effect of hemodiafiltration versus hemodialysis on the long-term progression of the arteriosclerotic process and discuss the potential implications that this effect may have in the choice of the most appropriate dialytic modality for ESRD patients.

2. Arterial stiffness in dialysis patients

Acceleration of the arteriosclerotic process is the typical feature of arterial remodeling in ESRD. Aortic and carotid-artery stiffness is significantly higher in ESRD patients than in age-, sex-, and BP-matched controls with normal renal function [15]. Among dialysis patients, arteriosclerotic process is a pathophysiological continuum of structural alterations that begin from the early stages of renal impairment, with several studies showing a stepwise increase in arterial stiffness with advancing stage of chronic kidney disease (CKD) [16, 17]. Structural alterations related to arterial stiffening in ESRD include fibro-elastic intimal thickening, calcification of elastic lamellae, increased extracellular matrix deposition, elastynolysis and inflammation, increased collagen, and decreased elastic fiber content [4, 18, 19]. The mechanistic background of these arterial wall alterations is complex and not yet fully elucidated. Apart from the contribution of accumulated traditional cardiovascular risk factors, it is suggested that specific mechanistic pathways related to the ESRD status and renal replacement therapy may play a particular role in the progression of arteriosclerosis in this population. Some of the most important ESRD-specific mechanisms involved in the pathogenesis of arteriosclerosis include impaired mineral metabolism and elevated calcium-phosphate product, vascular calcification, excessive activation of the RAAS, endothelial dysfunction, inflammation, oxidative stress, and chronic volume overload [4, 18, 19]. Compared with traditional cardiovascular risk factors, these ESRD-specific pathways were shown to be stronger determinants of the progression of arteriosclerosis over time [20].

The main physiological role of the aorta and large conduit arteries is (i) to dampen the high-pressure oscillations generated from the intermittent LV ejection and (ii) to transform the cyclic blood flow in the aorta into a continuous capillary flow pattern required for perfusion of organs and tissues [4, 19, 21]. During systole, the stroke volume ejected by the left ventricle interacts with the elastic properties of the aorta to generate a pulse wave (incident or forward-traveling) that is propagated at a pulse wave velocity (PWV) that progressively increases across the arterial tree. Structure of the arterial system is normally characterized by progressive increase in arterial wall stiffness from the ascending aorta to the peripheral muscular-type arteries (so-called stiffness gradient) [4, 19, 21]. Impendence mismatches at the transition between these segments generate pulse wave reflections. These reflected waves travel from the periphery back to the ascending aorta (backward-traveling reflected wave), opposing pulsatile energy transmission downstream to microcirculation. In young subjects with elastic central arteries, this process is coupled with slower pulse wave propagation and the overlap of the incident and reflected waves in the ascending aorta occurs in late systole or early diastole. This phenomenon results in rise of diastolic aortic pressure, favoring coronary perfusion during diastole. Arteriosclerotic process, however, affects preferentially the wall of the aorta and large central arteries, reversing the normal stiffness gradient between central and peripheral arterial segments [22]. In conditions of accelerated arterial stiffness, such as ESRD, there is premature arrival of reflected waves back to the ascending aorta, during systole rather than diastole [4, 19, 21]. This results in augmentation of central aortic systolic pressure, thereby increasing cardiac after load and promoting adverse myocardial remodeling toward fibrosis and hypertrophy. In addition, greater pulsatile energy transmission from macro- to microcirculation promotes microvascular damage in peripheral organs and tissues (**Figure 1**) [4, 19, 21].

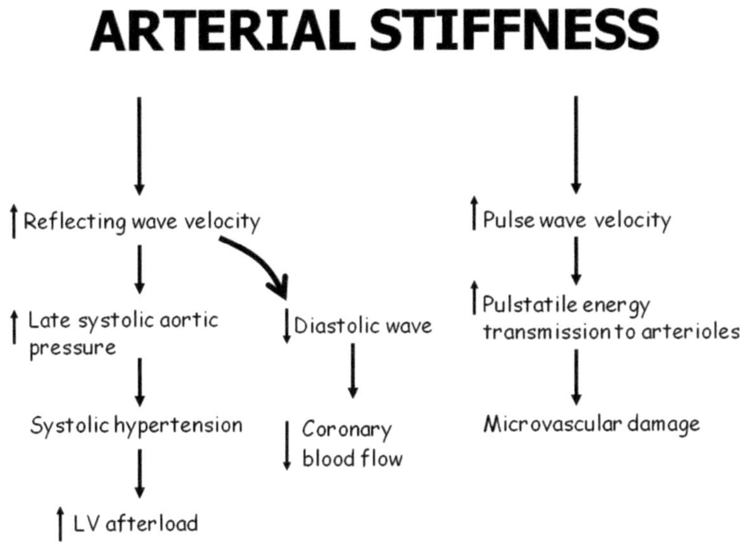

Figure 1. Pathophysiological role of increased arterial stiffness in ESRD.

The close pathophysiological association of arterial stiffness with promotion of end-organ damage is in line with a strong epidemiological association of increased arterial stiffness with worse cardiovascular outcomes. Among dialysis patients, prospective observational studies have for long-connected higher aortic PWV with increased risk of all-cause and cardiovascular mortality independently from other cardiovascular risk factors [7]. In the first study conducted in the late 1990s in a cohort of 241 hemodialysis patients prospectively followed for a mean period of 6 years, Blacher et al. [6] showed that the fully adjusted odds ratio (OR) for aortic PWV > 12.0 versus PWV < 9.4 m/s was 5.4 [95% confidence intervals (CIs): 2.4–11.9] for all-cause mortality and 5.9 (95% CI: 2.3–15.5) for cardiovascular mortality [6]. The strong prognostic association between aortic PWV and cardiovascular outcomes was confirmed in several subsequent cohorts of hemodialysis patients [15, 23]. Similarly to patients receiving hemodialysis, more recent observational studies have demonstrated the strong and independent prognostic significance of arterial stiffness in the whole spectrum of CKD, showing that aortic PWV is an independent predictor of mortality in patients receiving peritoneal dialysis [24] in renal transplant recipients [25] and in patients with CKD not yet on dialysis [26]. Most importantly, regression of arterial stiffness in response to BP-lowering was shown to be associated with improvement in survival [9], providing evidence that arterial stiffness is not simply a risk predictor, but a true cardiovascular risk factor in the dialysis population.

3. Studies comparing the effect of hemodiafiltration versus hemodialysis on arterial stiffness

Uremic toxin accumulation, particularly retention of protein-bound solutes and middle-weight molecules as a result of their inadequate clearance through conservative dialytic modalities, is proposed to play a prominent role in promoting vascular atherosclerosis and pathogenesis of cardiovascular disease among dialysis patients. In support of this notion, background and clinical studies have shown that accumulation of *p*-cresol and indoxyl sulfate, two protein-bound uremic toxins, acts as a triggering factor for the expression of pro-inflammatory cytokines and adhesion molecules, induces shedding of endothelial microparticles, and disrupts the nitric oxide signaling pathway [27–29]. Importantly, in recent prospective observational studies, high concentrations of both *p*-cresol and indoxyl sulfate in hemodialysis patients have been associated with increased risk of cardiovascular morbidity and mortality independently from other traditional cardiovascular risk factors [30–32].

Hemodiafiltration is a dialytic modality that uses a combination of convective transport and diffusion to enhance the removal of middle-to-high molecular weight solutes in comparison with standard hemodialysis [33, 34]. In some clinical studies, enhanced middle-molecule clearance achieved through convective dialytic modalities was shown to be associated with improvement in phosphate control, better preservation of intradialytic hemodynamic stability, as well as, with a number of beneficial actions on vasculature, such as reduction in circulating markers of vascular inflammation and oxidative stress and improvement in flow-mediated endothelium-dependent vasodilatation [11–14, 35]. These beneficial effects of hemodiafiltration on the vasculature have generated the hypothesis that switching ESRD patients from conventional hemodialysis to high-efficiency hemodiafiltration may be a therapeutic maneuver with potential advantages in causing regression of arterial stiffness. This hypothesis was tested in a number of clinical studies summarized in **Table 1** and discussed in detail below.

Author	Year	n	Patient characteristics	Design	Intervention	Follow-up (months)	Change in arterial stiffness over time	Overall effect
Beerenhout et al. [35]	2005	40	ESRD patients treated with thrice-weekly low-flux HD	RCT	Pre-dilution on-line HDF versus low-flux HD	12	Aortic PWV increased similarly over time in both dialytic modalities (HDF: 12 ± 5 versus 13 ± 5 m/s; HD: 12 ± 3 versus 13 ± 5 m/s)	Neutral
Bellien et al. [37]	2014	42	ESRD patients treated with thrice-weekly high-flux HD	RCT	Post-dilution on-line HDF versus high-flux HD	4	Carotid artery distensibility was increased in the on-line HDF group, but not in the HD group (between group difference: $-6.7\ kPa^{-1} \times 10^{-3}$, 95% CI: −9.9 to $-3.5\ kPa^{-1} \times 10^{-3}$, P = 0.048)	Better

Author	Year	n	Patient characteristics	Design	Intervention	Follow-up (months)	Change in arterial stiffness over time	Overall effect
Mostovaya et al. [39]	2014	189	ESRD patients participating in the CONTRAST trial	RCT	Post-dilution on-line HDF versus low-flux HD	36	Aortic PWV remained unchanged over time with both dialytic modalities (annual rate of PWV change: HDF group: −0.01, 95% CI: −0.41 to 0.40 m/s/year; HD group: −0.04, 95% CI: −0.31 to 0.23 m/s/year; p value HDF versus HD: 0.89)	Neutral
Charitaki et al. [38]	2014	289	ESRD patients on maintenance HD	Observational	69 patients on low-flux HD versus 78 patients switched from low-flux HD to HDF versus 142 patients on HDF	6	Aortic PWV increased over time in the low-flux HD group (9.5 ± 1.9 versus 10.2 ± 2.2 m/s, $p < 0.01$) as well as in the HD to HDF group (9.4 ± 1.9 versus 10.1 ± 2.2 m/s, $p < 0.01$), but remained constant in the HDF group (9.9 ± 2.1 versus 10.1 ± 2.2 m/s)	Better
Georgianos et al. [36]	2014	48	ESRD patients on maintenance HD	Observational	HDF versus low-flux HD	Single dialysis session	Aortic PWV remained unchanged from pre- to postdialysis either with HDF or with low-flux HD (HDF: 9.3 ± 0.5 versus 9.4 ± 0.5 m/s, p = 0.686 low-flux HD: 9.1 ± 0.4 versus 8.9 ± 0.4 m/s, p = 0.396)	Neutral

HD, hemodialysis; RCT, randomized controlled trial.

Table 1. Prospective studies comparing the effect of hemodiafiltration versus standard hemodialysis on arterial stiffness.

3.1. Acute effects of hemodiafiltration on arterial stiffness

In a nested case-control design, Georgianos et al. [36] compared the acute changes in aortic PWV from pre- to postdialysis in 24 ESRD patients receiving hemodiafiltration and in 24 age-

and sex-matched controls receiving low-flux hemodialysis. Aortic PWV was not significantly changed from pre- to postdialysis during both the first and second weekly dialysis sessions. These modest acute changes in aortic PWV from pre- to postdialysis were no different between the hemodiafiltration and low-flux hemodialysis groups in both dialysis sessions studied [36]. With regards to wave reflections, augmentation index and related parameters were significantly reduced from pre-to postdialysis in both dialysis sessions and patient groups. Similarly to aortic PWV, intradialytic reduction in wave reflection indices was no different between patients treated with hemodiafiltration and standard low-flux hemodialysis [36]. These findings suggest an acute intradialytic improvement in wave reflections from the periphery but not in aortic stiffness, an effect that was independent of the mode of dialysis. However, these comparable acute alterations in large-artery cushioning function do not necessarily prespecify the pattern of long-term progression of the arterial stiffness in patients treated with different dialytic modalities.

3.2. Long-term effects of hemodiafiltration on arterial stiffness

Studies evaluating the long-term effects of hemodiafiltration relative to hemodialysis on arterial structure and function provided contradictory results. Beerenhout et al. [35] randomized 40 ESRD patients treated with conventional low-flux hemodialysis to switch to high-efficiency pre-dilution on-line hemodiafiltration or to continue on the same dialytic modality. After 12 months of follow-up, aortic PWV increased similarly in both low-flux hemodialysis (12 ± 3 versus 13 ± 5 m/s) and on-line hemodiafiltration groups (12 ± 3 versus 13 ± 5 m/s). Notably, change in 48-h ambulatory systolic and diastolic BP and in LV mass index over time were also no difference between the two dialytic modalities [35]. Furthermore, on-line hemodiafiltration was not superior to low-flux hemodialysis in inhibiting the formation of advanced glycation end-products and reducing the circulating levels of asymmetric dimethylarginine (ADMA) and markers of oxidative stress or total anti-oxidant capacity. In a subsequent study, 42 ESRD patients were randomly assigned to switch from high-flux conventional hemodialysis to high-efficiency post-dilution on-line hemodiafiltration or to remain on high-flux hemodialysis for a mean follow-up period of 4 months [37]. Arterial stiffness assessed with the use of the distensibility co-efficient of the common carotid artery was improved in the on-line hemodiafiltration group, but not in the high-flux conventional hemodialysis group (between-group difference: $-6.7\ kPa^{-1} \times 10^{-3}$, 95% CI: -9.9 to $-3.5\ kPa^{-1} \times 10^{-3}$, $p = 0.048$) [37]. Improvement in carotid artery distensibility was accompanied by a significant improvement in Kt/V urea, predialysis levels of β2-microglobulin, circulating levels of ADMA and tumor necrosis factor (TNF)-a, and brachial artery flow-mediated endothelium-dependent vasodilatation. In a multiple regression analysis model, hemodiafiltration-induced improvement in conduit artery endothelial dysfunction and stiffness was associated with the changes in Kt/V urea and predialysis levels of β2-microglobulin, suggesting that enhanced clearance of middle-to-high molecular weight solutes is one factor potentially contributing to the beneficial effect of hemodiafiltration on large-artery stiffness.

A beneficial effect of hemodiafiltration on arterial stiffness is supported by another observational study, in which aortic PWV measurements were performed 6 months apart in three different groups of ESRD patients [38]. The first group consisted of 69 ESRD patients receiving conventional low-flux hemodialysis, the second group consisted of 78 ESRD patients who were switched from low-flux hemodialysis to on-line hemodiafiltration, and the third group included 142 ESRD patients receiving long-term renal replacement therapy with on-line hemodiafiltration. Over the 6-month observational period, a significant increase in aortic PWV was noted in those patients treated with hemodialysis (9.5 ± 1.9 versus 10.2 ± 2.2 m/s, $p < 0.01$) as well as in those switched from hemodialysis to hemodiafiltration (9.4 ± 1.9 versus 10.1 ± 2.2 m/s, $p < 0.01$); in contrast, aortic PWV remained unchanged in the group of hemodiafiltration (9.9 ± 2.1 versus 10.1 ± 2.2 m/s) [38]. The most important finding of this study was that aortic PWV remained constant during follow-up only in those patients receiving long-term treatment with hemodiafiltration, whereas aortic PWV increased in patients who were switched from hemodialysis to hemodiafiltration. This observation could be interpreted in two different ways: either the 6-month-long therapy with hemodiafiltration might be inadequate in order to modify the arterial wall structure and stiffness, or aortic PWV increased in those patients switched to hemodiafiltration due to a carry-on effect of previous long-term therapy with conventional hemodialysis.

The above beneficial impact of hemodiafiltration in causing regression of arterial stiffness was not confirmed in a recent subanalysis of 189 prevalent dialysis patients participating in the CONvective TRAnsport STudy (CONTRAST) trial [39]. In this study, ESRD patients receiving conventional low-flux hemodialysis were randomly assigned in a 1:1 ratio for treatment with on-line hemodiafiltration or continuation of low-flux hemodialysis for a mean follow-up period of 36 months. Median aortic PWV at baseline was 9.8 m/s (interquartile range: 7.5–12.0 m/s). Aortic PWV was not significantly changed over time, and the annual rate of PWV change had no difference between the on-line hemodiafiltration and hemodialysis groups (hemodiafiltration group: −0.01 m/s/year, 95% CIs: −0.41 to 0.40 m/s/year; hemodialysis group: −0.04 m/s/year, 95% CI: −0.31 to 0.23 m/s/year; p value for the between-group comparison: 0.89) [39]. The absence of difference between the two dialytic modalities in the rate of PWV change was consistent across subgroups of age, sex, residual renal function, dialysis vintage, diabetes, and history of pre-existing cardiovascular disease. Of note, the annual rate of PWV change had once again no difference between the two dialytic modalities regardless of the convection volume used for on-line hemodiafiltration (convection volume <18.9 L/session: 0.37 m/s/year; 95% CIs: −0.25 to 0.98 m/s/year, $p = 0.23$; convection volume >18.9 L/session: −0.01 m/s/year; 95% CIs: −0.59 to 0.57, $p = 0.99$) [39].

4. Studies comparing the effect of hemodiafiltration versus hemodialysis on mortality

The above contradictory results of clinical studies that evaluated the comparative effectiveness of hemodialfiltration versus standard hemodialysis in causing regression of arterial stiffness

http://dx.doi.org/10.5772/63369

are in line with the uncertain superiority of hemodiafiltration on mortality across large-scaled randomized controlled trials that included "hard" cardiovascular outcomes as primary endpoints. For example, in the primary analysis of the aforementioned CONTRAST study [40], 714 ESRD patients were randomly assigned to switch from low-flux hemodialysis to on-line hemodiafiltration or continue renal replacement therapy with low-flux hemodialysis. After a mean follow-up period of 3 years, incidence of all-cause mortality [Hazard Ratio (HR): 0.95; 95% CIs: 0.75–1.20] and occurrence of fatal and non-fatal cardiovascular events (HR: 1.07; 95% CIs: 0.83–1.39) were not different between the two dialytic modalities [40]. The subsequent Turkish on-line hemodiafiltration (OL-HDF) study enrolled 782 ESRD patients receiving standard thrice-weekly hemodialysis who were randomly assigned in a 1:1 ratio to post-dilution on-line hemodiafiltration or high-flux conventional hemodialysis [41]. Over a mean follow-up period of 22.7 ± 10.9 months, the occurrence of the composite primary outcome of all-cause mortality and non-fatal cardiovascular event was identical in both study arms (event-free survival of 77.6% in hemodiafiltration versus 74.8% in the high-flux group, P = 0.28) [41]. Contrary to the above results, the Estudio de Supervivencia de Hemodiafiltración On-Line (ESHOL) study supports the notion that on-line hemodiafiltration is superior over hemodialysis in reducing all-cause and cardiovascular mortality [42]. In this open-label, randomized controlled trial, 906 prevalent hemodialysis patients were randomly assigned either to switch to high-efficiency post-dilution on-line hemodiafiltration or to remain on standard low-flux hemodialysis. Switching from low-flux hemodialysis to on-line hemodiafiltration was associated with a 30% risk reduction for all-cause mortality (HR: 0.70; 95% CI: 0.53–0.92), 33% risk reduction for cardiovascular mortality (HR: 0.67; 95% CIs: 0.44–1.02) and 55% risk reduction for infection-related mortality (HR: 0.45; 95% CIs: 0.21–0.96) [42].

5. Conclusion

In summary, the currently available evidence from observational and randomized clinical studies does not conclusively support a clear superiority of hemodiafiltration versus standard hemodialysis in improving arterial compliance. The contradictory results of clinical studies with respect to PWV, a surrogate cardiovascular risk factor, are in line with the uncertain survival benefit of convective dialytic modalities in large-scaled clinical trials evaluating "hard" cardiovascular outcomes. Additional research efforts are urgently warranted to fully elucidate the comparative effectiveness of hemodiafiltration versus conventional hemodialysis on arterial stiffness attenuation. In the meantime, we believe that dialysis treatment optimization is undoubtedly one useful tool toward cardiovascular risk reduction for patients receiving maintenance hemodialysis.

Author details

Panagiotis I. Georgianos[1], Evangelia Dounousi[2], Theodoros Eleftheriadis[1] and Vassilios Liakopoulos[1*]

*Address all correspondence to: liakopul@otenet.gr

1 Division of Nephrology and Hypertension, 1st Department of Internal Medicine, AHEPA Hospital, Aristotle University of Thessaloniki, Thessaloniki, Greece

2 Department of Nephrology, Medical School, University of Ioannina, Ioannina, Greece

References

[1] Go AS, Chertow GM, Fan D, McCulloch CE, Hsu CY. Chronic kidney disease and the risks of death, cardiovascular events, and hospitalization. *N Engl J Med* 2004;351(13): 1296–305.

[2] Tonelli M, Wiebe N, Culleton B, et al. Chronic kidney disease and mortality risk: a systematic review. *J Am Soc Nephrol* 2006;17(7):2034–47.

[3] 2013 USRDS annual data report: cardiovascular disease. 2:252–262.

[4] Laurent S, Cockcroft J, Van Bortel L, et al. Expert consensus document on arterial stiffness: methodological issues and clinical applications. *Eur Heart J* 2006;27(21):2588–605.

[5] Taal MW. Arterial stiffness in chronic kidney disease: an update. *Curr Opin Nephrol Hypertens* 2014;23(2):169–73.

[6] Blacher J, Guerin AP, Pannier B, Marchais SJ, Safar ME, London GM. Impact of aortic stiffness on survival in end-stage renal disease. *Circulation* 1999;99(18):2434–9.

[7] Georgianos PI, Sarafidis PA, Lasaridis AN. Arterial stiffness: a novel cardiovascular risk factor in kidney disease patients. *Curr Vasc Pharmacol*;13(2):229–38.

[8] Chirinos JA, Townsend RR. Reducing arterial stiffness in CKD: revising the paradigms. *Clin J Am Soc Nephrol*;10(4):547–50.

[9] Guerin AP, Blacher J, Pannier B, Marchais SJ, Safar ME, London GM. Impact of aortic stiffness attenuation on survival of patients in end-stage renal failure. *Circulation* 2001;103(7):987–92.

[10] Blankestijn PJ, Ledebo I, Canaud B. Hemodiafiltration: clinical evidence and remaining questions. *Kidney Int* 2010;77(7):581–7.

[11] Locatelli F, Altieri P, Andrulli S, et al. Hemofiltration and hemodiafiltration reduce intradialytic hypotension in ESRD. *J Am Soc Nephrol* 2010;21(10):1798–807.

[12] Oates T, Pinney JH, Davenport A. Haemodiafiltration versus high-flux haemodialysis: effects on phosphate control and erythropoietin response. *Am J Nephrol* 2011;33(1):70–5.

[13] Ward RA, Schmidt B, Hullin J, Hillebrand GF, Samtleben W. A comparison of on-line hemodiafiltration and high-flux hemodialysis: a prospective clinical study. *J Am Soc Nephrol* 2000;11(12):2344–50.

[14] Wizemann V, Lotz C, Techert F, Uthoff S. On-line haemodiafiltration versus low-flux haemodialysis. A prospective randomized study. *Nephrol Dial Transplant* 2000;15(Suppl 1):43–8.

[15] Pannier B, Guerin AP, Marchais SJ, Safar ME, London GM. Stiffness of capacitive and conduit arteries: prognostic significance for end-stage renal disease patients. *Hypertension* 2005;45(4):592–6.

[16] Georgianos PI, Sarafidis PA, Liakopoulos V. Arterial stiffness: a novel risk factor for kidney injury progression? *Am J Hypertens* 2015;28(8):958–65.

[17] Kimoto E, Shoji T, Shinohara K, et al. Regional arterial stiffness in patients with type 2 diabetes and chronic kidney disease. *J Am Soc Nephrol* 2006;17(8):2245–52.

[18] Briet M, Burns KD. Chronic kidney disease and vascular remodelling: molecular mechanisms and clinical implications. *Clin Sci (Lond)* 2012;123(7):399–416.

[19] London G, Covic A, Goldsmith D, et al. Arterial aging and arterial disease: interplay between central hemodynamics, cardiac work, and organ flow-implications for CKD and cardiovascular disease. *Kidney Int Suppl* 2011;1(1):10–2.

[20] Utescu MS, Couture V, Mac-Way F, et al. Determinants of progression of aortic stiffness in hemodialysis patients: a prospective longitudinal study. *Hypertension* 2013;62(1): 154–60.

[21] O'Rourke MF. Wave travel and reflection in the arterial system. *J Hypertens Suppl* 1999;17(5):S45–S47.

[22] Kimoto E, Shoji T, Shinohara K, et al. Preferential stiffening of central over peripheral arteries in type 2 diabetes. *Diabetes* 2003;52(2):448–52.

[23] London GM, Safar ME, Pannier B. Arterial aging in ESRD: structural, hemodynamic, and mortality implications. *J Am Soc Nephrol* doi: 10.1681/ASN.2015060617 2015.

[24] Szeto CC, Kwan BC, Chow KM, Leung CB, Law MC, Li PK. Prognostic value of arterial pulse wave velocity in peritoneal dialysis patients. *Am J Nephrol* 2012;35(2):127–33.

[25] Mitchell A, Opazo SA, Kos M, Witzke O, Kribben A, Nurnberger J. Pulse wave velocity predicts mortality in renal transplant patients. *Eur J Med Res* 2010;15(10):452–5.

[26] Karras A, Haymann JP, Bozec E, et al. Large artery stiffening and remodeling are independently associated with all-cause mortality and cardiovascular events in chronic kidney disease. *Hypertension* 2012;60(6):1451–7.

[27] Dou L, Burtey S. The harmful effect of indoxyl sulfate on neovascularization in chronic kidney disease. *Kidney Int* 2016;89(3):532–4.

[28] Tumur Z, Niwa T. Indoxyl sulfate inhibits nitric oxide production and cell viability by inducing oxidative stress in vascular endothelial cells. *Am J Nephrol* 2009;29(6):551–7.

[29] Wu IW, Hsu KH, Lee CC, et al. p-Cresyl sulphate and indoxyl sulphate predict progression of chronic kidney disease. *Nephrol Dial Transplant* 2011;26(3):938–47.

[30] Cao XS, Chen J, Zou JZ, et al. Association of indoxyl sulfate with heart failure among patients on hemodialysis. *Clin J Am Soc Nephrol* 2015;10(1):111–9.

[31] Meijers BK, Bammens B, De MB, Verbeke K, Vanrenterghem Y, Evenepoel P. Free p-cresol is associated with cardiovascular disease in hemodialysis patients. *Kidney Int* 2008;73(10):1174–80.

[32] Meijers BK, Claes K, Bammens B, et al. p-Cresol and cardiovascular risk in mild-to-moderate kidney disease. *Clin J Am Soc Nephrol* 2010;5(7):1182–9.

[33] Bammens B, Evenepoel P, Verbeke K, Vanrenterghem Y. Removal of the protein-bound solute p-cresol by convective transport: a randomized crossover study. *Am J Kidney Dis* 2004;44(2):278–85.

[34] Cornelis T, van der Sande FM, Eloot S, et al. Acute hemodynamic response and uremic toxin removal in conventional and extended hemodialysis and hemodiafiltration: a randomized crossover study. *Am J Kidney Dis* 2014;64(2):247–56.

[35] Beerenhout CH, Luik AJ, Jeuken-Mertens SG, et al. Pre-dilution on-line haemofiltration vs low-flux haemodialysis: a randomized prospective study. *Nephrol Dial Transplant* 2005;20(6):1155–63.

[36] Georgianos PI, Sarafidis PA, Karpetas A, et al. Hemodiafiltration does not have additional benefits over hemodialysis on arterial stiffness, wave reflections and central aortic pressures. *Blood Purif* 2014;37(1):18–26.

[37] Bellien J, Freguin-Bouilland C, Joannides R, et al. High-efficiency on-line haemodiafiltration improves conduit artery endothelial function compared with high-flux haemodialysis in end-stage renal disease patients. *Nephrol Dial Transplant* 2014;29(2):414–22.

[38] Charitaki E, Davenport A. Does hemodiafiltration reduce vascular stiffness measured by aortic pulse wave velocity compared with high-flux hemodialysis? *Hemodial Int* 2014;18(2):391–5.

[39] Mostovaya IM, Bots ML, van den Dorpel MA, et al. A randomized trial of hemodiafiltration and change in cardiovascular parameters. *Clin J Am Soc Nephrol* 2014;9(3):520–6.

[40] Grooteman MP, van den Dorpel MA, Bots ML, et al. Effect of online hemodiafiltration on all-cause mortality and cardiovascular outcomes. *J Am Soc Nephrol* 2012;23(6):1087–96.

[41] Ok E, Asci G, Toz H, et al. Mortality and cardiovascular events in online haemodiafiltration (OL-HDF) compared with high-flux dialysis: results from the Turkish OL-HDF Study. *Nephrol Dial Transplant* 2013;28(1):192–202.

[42] Maduell F, Moreso F, Pons M, et al. High-efficiency postdilution online hemodiafiltration reduces all-cause mortality in hemodialysis patients. *J Am Soc Nephrol* 2013;24(3):487–97.

Chapter 5

Effectiveness of Ultrafiltration in Patients with Congestive Heart Failure

Luai Alhazmi, Abdulelah Nuqali, Ankush Moza and Mujeeb Sheikh

Additional information is available at the end of the chapter

http://dx.doi.org/10.5772/63393

Abstract

Among all cardiac diseases, congestive heart failure (CHF) is the leading cause of patient rehospitalization. Fluid overload and lung congestion are the major reasons for these recurrent admissions. This disease can be associated with worsening renal function, a phenomenon called cardiorenal syndrome (CRS), which is challenging to manage. Conventional diuretic therapy of both CRS and diuretic resistance has offered limited efficacy. Compared with conventional therapy, hemodiafiltration (HDF) has shown promising results for fluid removal in some clinical trials, with inconclusive effects on all-cause mortality and rehospitalizations. Nonetheless, the results are inconsistent because of the high heterogeneity among these studies. In this chapter, we shed light on the role of different methods of ultrafiltration, including peritoneal ultrafiltration, sustained slow efficiency dialysis, and HDF, in the management of CHF, and review the current literature.

Keywords: congestive heart failure, cardiorenal syndrome, peritoneal ultrafiltration, sustained low efficiency dialysis, hemodiafiltration

1. Introduction

Congestive heart failure (CHF), sometimes called chronic heart failure or simply heart failure, is a disease that affects a patient's everyday life and can have deleterious effects on both physical and mental well-being [1–3]. Patients with CHF have a worse health-related quality of life than those with many other chronic diseases, such as chronic obstructive pulmonary disease, hypertension, diabetes mellitus, and myocardial infarction [3, 4]. Moreover, rehospitalizations are a major concern among these patients, their families, and their health service providers. CHF causes the highest rehospitalization rate among all chronic diseases, reaching up to 27% [5]. Patients with CHF have a poor prognosis, with a 1-year survival rate that is comparable or worse than that for common neoplasms such as prostatic or breast malignancies. Stewart et al. showed that the median survival time for patients with CHF was 16 months with 25% 5-year survival rate [6, 7]. Despite all advances in the management of CHF, it is still the leading cause of mortality among cardiac diseases [8, 9]. Fluid overload and lung congestion are the most recurrent cause of admissions in these patients [10]. Almost 50% of them are discharged with residual congestion, and most rehospitalizations occur in patients who are diuretic resistant [11]. Diuretic resistance, in which patients with CHF have reduced diuresis and natriuresis in response to diuretics, causes higher mortality and rehospitalizations [10, 12, 13]. CHF is also associated with cardiorenal syndrome (CRS), a condition in which renal function worsens and is challenging to manage [14]. Conventional diuretic therapy of both CRS and diuretic resistance has shown limited efficacy with no robust data on efficacy in terms of well-designed randomized clinical controlled trials [15, 16]. However, hemodiafiltration (HDF), isotonic fluid replacement through positive hydrostatic pressure, has recently emerged as an alternative or last resort for these complex patients. The aim of this physiological approach is to decrease neurohumoral activation, which in turn curbs the vicious cycle leading to cardiac and renal insult [17, 18]. Some promising results have been reported in initial studies, but the data conflict and are inconclusive. As a result, no clinical guidelines to date have adopted HDF as an alternative to diuretic therapy [10, 19–22].

2. Diuretic resistance and CRS syndrome

No specified definition is available for diuretic resistance, as it is the outcome of treatment and not a pathological condition in itself. The efficacy of loop diuretics can be evaluated as a measure of urine output, change in weight, and balance in net fluid [23]. Patients unable to meet their needs for decongestion despite high doses of loop diuretics are generally labeled as diuretic resistant. Some current studies have reported the efficacy of diuretics in terms of clinical outcomes in patients with CHF [24–31]. Although these studies used different methods and metrics, the outcomes were similar in all: patients with diuretic resistance showed poor outcomes compared with those without diuretic resistance. Even after correcting for glomerular filtration rate (GFR), a strong correlation between worse clinical results and diuretic resistance was observed, showing that the efficacy of diuretics and the GFR each have a different impact on clinical outcomes. GFR is a good indicator of the kidney's clearance ability. When this rate is normal, the renal tubules are able to maintain homeostasis of electrolytes and euvolemia. Even if the GFR is reduced to up to 20 mL/min, usually 28.8 L of fluid is filtered, and sodium excretion is about 4000 mEq. The metrics used in current studies for diuretic efficacy are indirectly related to the effectiveness of loop diuretics for sodium excretion. Consequently, these metrics indicate a better prognosis than does the GFR in terms of the kidneys achieving euvolemia.

Several studies that used different metrics tried to establish a correlation between efficacy of diuretics and heart failure-related clinical outcomes. In the case of patients having reduced diuretic efficacy, Testani et al. [24] found high mortality rates even after correcting for diuretic dose and fluid output. Valente et al. [25] and Voors et al. [31] observed increased death and rehospitalization rates associated with diuretic resistance in heart failure at 60 days, whereas Ter Maaten et al. [28] reported similar outcomes at 30-day follow-up. After correcting for the GFR, Verbrugge et al. [29] and Singh et al. [26] reported higher death and rehospitalization rates related to diuretic resistance.

On the contrary, CRS is a condition that becomes apparent from a decrease in the GFR and acts as a barrier to the treatment of CHF by limiting the renal function [32]. At first, a decrease in blood flow in the kidney was considered to cause a low GFR, but recently a number of studies have shown that cardiorenal interactions have several complex mechanisms, some of which may be reversible. In a commonly used classification given by Ronco and colleagues [33], CRS is grouped into four types: type 1 is characterized by acute heart failure, leading to acute kidney injury; type 2 involves chronic cardiac impairment such as CHF, resulting in chronic kidney disease; type 3 is a result of primary kidney function impairments, resulting in acute cardiac impairment that may become evident as heart failure; and type 4 involves chronic cardiac impairments influenced primarily by primary chronic kidney disease such as uremic cardiomyopathy. A further type 5 CRS involves systemic disorders of the chronic or acute type such as sepsis; diabetes causes both cardiac and renal dysfunction.

Acute CRS is a reflection of worsening renal function in patients with CHF [34]. CRS is found in 25–33% of all patients with acute decompensated heart failure (ADHF) [35, 36]. Extrarenal hemodynamic changes, cellular dysregulation, neurohormonal activation, and intrarenal microvascular and oxidative stress underlie acute CRS [34, 37]. In a few cases, intravenous diuretic-mediated renal injury is responsible for worsening renal function [16, 38, 37]. Other proposed mechanisms of CRS pathophysiology include neurohumoral adaptations, reduced renal perfusions, elevated venous pressure, and dysfunction of the right ventricle [39, 40].

3. Peritoneal ultrafiltration (pUF)

In advanced stages of CHF, a decline in renal function can often be seen, consistent with type 2 CRS (CRS-2). Several therapies have been evaluated for this group of patients; however, the optimal therapy for "chronic" CRS remains elusive. It is believed that peritoneal ultrafiltration (pUF) may lead to improvement in the clinical function of these patients, with a reduction in the number of hospitalizations.

A study performed on patients without end-stage renal disease evaluated the efficacy of pUF in the treatment of chronic refractory heart failure (HF) [41]. For this evaluation, 39 consecutive patients with end-stage CHF and stable CRS-2 were given ambulatory pUF and prospectively followed for 1 year. The primary end point was all-cause hospitalization. Mortality, treatment changes, and weight changes with New York Heart Association (NYHA) functional class and quality of life were considered as the secondary end points. Compared with the control group, who received standard treatment, in the pUF group, there was a reduction in the number of

1-year hospitalization days ($p = 0.07$). However, the 1-year mortality was found to be 33% in the pUF group and 23% in the control cohort, although this result was not statistically significant. In comparison to standard medical treatment, pUF was found to significantly improve volume overload ($p < 0.05$), the NYHA functional class ($p < 0.001$), and mental health ($p < 0.05$) of the patients. Furthermore, in the pUF group, the hospitalization days for all causes, including cardiovascular incidents, were significantly reduced during the interim periods ($p < 0.05$ and $p < 0.001$, respectively).

Another study evaluated pUF in patients with severe HF that was refractory to aggressive drug therapy [42]. Treatment with pUF was considered in these patients, as they had been hospitalized at least three times in the preceding year for ADHF that had required extracorporeal UF. This study comprised 48 patients; of those, 30 received one nocturnal icodextrin exchange, 5 received two daily exchanges, and the remaining 13 received two to four sessions per week of automated peritoneal dialysis (PD). In the first year of therapy, renal function remained stable with a decline in pulmonary artery systolic pressure to 40 ± 6.09 mmHg from 45.5 ± 9.18 mmHg ($p = 0.03$). At the same time, significant improvement was noted in the NYHA functional status. Furthermore, patient hospitalizations decreased to 11 ± 17 days/patient-year from 43 ± 33 days/patient-year seen in the preceding year, which was before the onset of PUF treatment ($p < 0.001$). Thus, this study confirms the efficacy of PUF treatment in elderly patients with chronic HF.

Recently, a systematic review conducted to evaluate the efficacy of PD in patients with refractory CHF identified 21 studies from 13 countries [43]. This review comprised 673 patients and suggested that in patients with refractory CHF, PD can be an effective and safe treatment option, leading to improved heart function and weight control. It also reported that PD can reduce patient hospitalization days without any progressive worsening of renal function. The rates of PD complications such as peritonitis were also found to be acceptable.

4. Sustained low-efficiency dialysis (SLED) in patients with CHF

Sustained low-efficiency dialysis (SLED), or sustained low-efficiency daily dialysis (SLEDD), is a conventional hemodialysis that is performed over a longer period (6–12 h) of time using lower rates of blood flow (50–200 mL/min) and dialysate flow (200–400 mL/min). It is an alternative treatment in critically ill patients with affected kidney function [44–46], where fluid is removed slowly over longer time ensuring better hemodynamic stability [47]. This is in particular the case when the cost of HF/HDF is considered expensive. It combines the logistic advantages, the cost-effectiveness and the scheduling flexibility of the intermittent dialysis, and the hemodynamic stability of continuous renal replacement therapy with fewer side effects during the fluid removal [48]. There is still a limited clinical data in the literature on the effectiveness of SLED in patients with CHF. However, Iorio et al.'s experience suggested that SLED is an alternative treatment for acute dialysis in patients with diuretic resistant systolic CHF [49]. Violi et al. mentioned that the SLED as an alternative treatment is the most indicated in NYHA class IV CHF [50].

http://dx.doi.org/10.5772/63393

5. Hemodiafiltration in a nutshell

Dialysis refers to diffusive clearance. During dialysis, low-molecular weight solutes such as sodium and potassium move down their concentration gradient. The solute must be of appropriate size to pass through a semi-permeable membrane. By passing fluid across the membrane countercurrent to blood flow, equilibration of plasma and dialysate solute concentrations occur. This process may remove or add solute to the plasma water space depending upon the relative concentrations in dialysate and plasma. At the same time, water will also move along a gradient, in this case the osmolar or osmotic gradient, in effect "following" the solute. Diffusive clearance is more effective at removal of small solute, such as serum ions and urea, than for larger solutes.

Hemofiltration (HF) or ultrafiltration (UF) refers to convective clearance. The difference from dialysis is that pressure gradient rather than concentration gradient has its main effect on water movement. Solute movement is secondary and in conjunction with water. The transmembrane pressure difference can be adjusted as needed to remove water from the body down a pressure gradient. The flow of plasma water "drags" solute with it in the formation of ultrafiltrate. UF or HF is far superior for fluid clearance than diffusive clearance, and small solute clearance is almost identical. Slow continuous ultrafiltration (SCUF) is a term used for removing isotonic plasma water, which is indicated in patients with fluid overload such as those with CHF.

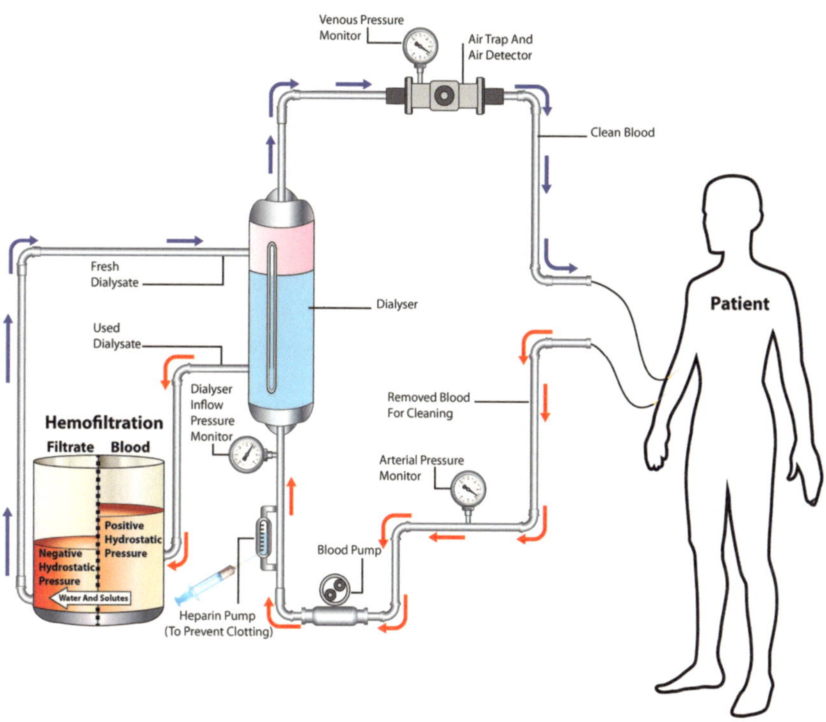

Figure 1. Principle of hemodiafiltration.

Hemodiaflitraion refers to a combination of convective and diffusive therapies. An example is the use of continuous venovenous hemodiafiltration (CVVHDF) in critically ill patients. It constitutes lower blood flow rate and slower fluid removal which may cause less hemodynamic instability in a hypotensive critically ill patient [51].

The setup for HDF requires a double-lumen central venous catheter, a peristaltic pump, and a filter inserted into a venovenous extracorporeal circuit [52] (**Figure 1**). Negative pressure generated by the pump allows blood circulation in the circuit, starting from the central vein and returning to the patient through the filter. Pore fibers of the filter keep water and small particles separated from blood through convective transport. Plasma water flow makes the blood concentration transient, eventually causing intravascular refilling while transferring liquids from the outer to the inner vascular space, thus safeguarding the circulating volume.

After the dispatched intravascular fluid is replaced by extravascular fluid refilling, hypovolemia can be prevented, thus preventing hemodynamic worsening. According to previous reported studies, fluid removal through HDF has affirmative hemodynamic effects. A study was done on 24 patients with resistant CHF undergoing UF; blood gas analysis (in both systemic and pulmonary arteries), plasma volume changes, and plasma refilling rate were measured after every liter of plasma water removed; UF was performed safely without side effects or hemodynamic instability; and mean right atrial, pulmonary artery and wedge pressures progressively reduced during the procedure [18]. Heart rate and systemic vascular resistance did not increase, and other peripheral biochemical parameters did not worsen during UF. Cardiac output increased at the end of the procedure and, to a greater extent, 24 h later, in relation to the increase of stroke volume. Intravascular volume remained stable throughout the entire duration of the procedure, indicating that a proportional volume of fluid was refilled from the congested parenchyma. Thus, UF is associated with hemodynamic improvement. Fluid refilling from the over-hydrated interstitium is the major compensatory mechanism for intravascular fluid removal, and hypotension does not occur when plasma refilling rate is adequate to prevent hypovolemia.

When a patient in decompensated heart failure is treated with HDF, it is important to ensure that the amount of removed intravascular water is below the amount of the capillary refilling rate; otherwise, neurohumoral activation can lead the patient to hypotension and abnormal renal function [18]. Thus, the distinctive feature of HDF is its effectiveness in removing extravascular fluids without increasing or decreasing the circulating volume and in turn avoiding neurohormonal activation and its consequences [52]. Respiratory symptoms such as dyspnea and orthopnea can be improved not only by total fluid removal but also by improvement in lung mechanics, pulmonary gas exchange, interstitial edema, vascular congestion, etc. [53, 54]. The two strategies (mechanical and pharmacological) of fluid withdrawal can have different effects on intravascular volume, hemodynamics, neurohumoral activity, and other regulatory mechanisms, leading to differing clinical outcomes. The tonicity of the fluid removed by the two strategies is different (isotonic with ultrafiltration [UF] and hypotonic with loop diuretics) [52, 55, 56]. With HDF, intravascular volume can be preserved, whereas it can be reduced with loop diuretics. After HDF, a better water-salt balance can be achieved and maintained in the body, whereas rapid worsening of this balance to the baseline abnormal state can occur with loop diuretics. A number of pathophysiology-oriented studies have documented these concepts [18, 53, 57]. Still, some ambiguity remains regarding the exact mechanisms of HDF in treating CRS and diuretic resistance.

6. Overview of clinical trials on HDF

An Israeli study aimed to determine the appropriateness and safety of UF therapy in patients with CHF who were admitted to outpatient clinics between April and September 2013 [58]. HDF was used to treat several patients with chronic CHF with NYHA III-IV and diuretic resistance. A total of 38 courses of treatment were administered. The results showed that about 1982 mL of fluid was removed per course, and patients reported having a subjective feeling of improvement in symptoms. Another Singaporean retrospective study was conducted among 44 patients who were admitted to the hospital from October 2011 to July 2013 [59] for decompensated heart failure and diuretic resistance. The study authors concluded that HDF is an effective and safe treatment strategy that can ameliorate the health of diuretic-resistant Asian patients with decompensated CHF.

Therefore, HDF has proven to be an effective method for fluid removal. It is adjustable in terms of both fluid volumes and rates with no changes in the levels of serum electrolytes. However, despite the effectiveness of HDF in fluid removal, clinical studies have not discovered any clinical benefit of this method over diuretic therapy. Furthermore, compared with diuresis, HDF does not preserve renal function.

In February 2016, a published study compared the effectiveness of HDF and loop diuresis in patients with heart failure (HF) [60]. This study comprised 105 patients with HF who were receiving UF and 108 patients with HF who were receiving adjustable loop diuretics. The aim of the study was to compare the recurrence of HF in the two groups at 90-day follow-up. However, the small sample size provided inconclusive data, which could not be used to identify a significant difference between the two patient groups. The authors of this study reported that the first HF event within 90 days of hospital discharge was seen in 25% of patients who received adjustable UF and in 35% of patients who received adjustable loop diuretics. Furthermore, there were approximately 62 days leading to the first HF event in the 25% patient group and 34 days leading to this even in the 35% patient group. Despite the trend toward better results with HDF, this difference did not reach statistical significance (log rank p 1/4 0.106). The hazard ratio, which was found to be 0.663 (95% confidence interval [CI] 0.402 to 1.092), suggested a 37% lower risk of an HF event with adjustable UF compared with adjustable loop diuretic therapy, but this result was statistically insignificant. The results should be interpreted with caution, as the study was unilateral and was prematurely terminated by the sponsor.

Another study that included 188 patients investigated UF in CRS [37]. Half of the patients were given stepped pharmacological therapy, and the other half were treated with UF. The bivariate change of the serum creatinine level and body weight from baseline, calculated after 96 h, was the primary end point of the study. The patients were then followed for 60 days. After 96 h, patients undergoing stepped pharmacological therapy had superior renal function compared with that in patients receiving UF. A similar amount of weight loss was noted in both groups of patients. In addition, UF was found to be associated with a higher rate of adverse events.

For patients with CHF, UF is usually reserved for cases of renal failure or unresponsiveness to pharmacological therapy. To study the safety and effectiveness of UF in patients hospitalized with decompensated CHF, investigators conducted the relief for acutely fluid-overloaded patients with decompensated congestive heart failure (RAPID-CHF) trial. This study, the first randomized controlled trial to compare UF with medical therapy, comprised 40 subjects [61]. A single 8-h course of UF with peripherally inserted catheters, along with supportive care and treatment, was compared with supportive care only. Patients who received UF had a greater volume of fluid removal (median 4650 vs. 2838 mL, $p = 0.001$) and improved signs and symptoms of congestion. Treatment with UF was well tolerated by the patients and did not result in any major adverse effects such as hemodynamic and renal complications. Thus, as can be deduced from the study, early treatment with UF for patients with CHF is a feasible treatment option that is well tolerated and can result in significant weight loss and fluid removal.

Another study supporting the findings of the RAPID-CHF trial was the ultrafiltration versus intravenous diuretics for patients hospitalized for acute decompensated heart failure (UNLOAD) trial [62]. The purpose of this randomized controlled trial was to study the safety and effectiveness of early treatment with primary UF in patients with ADHF. The study comprised 200 subjects with two or more signs of hypervolemia. At 48 h after the onset of treatment, weight reduction (5.0 ± 3.1 vs. 3.1 ± 3.5 kg, $p = 0.001$) and net fluid loss (4.6 vs. 3.3 L. $p = 0.001$) were higher in patients who were receiving UF. Furthermore, compared with the patients who were receiving diuretic therapy, the UF group showed lower rates of rehospitalization (0.22 ± 0.54 vs. 0.46 ± 0.76) with fewer days of in-hospital stay (1.4 ± 4.2 days vs. 3.8 ± 8.5 days) and fewer unscheduled medical visits (21% vs. 44%) within 90 days of hospital discharge. Throughout the study, changes in serum creatinine levels were similar in both groups. Episodes of hypotension during the first 48 h after hospitalization were similar (4% vs. 3%) in both groups. Thus, the UNLOAD trial demonstrated that, in patients with ADHF, UF is a safe treatment choice that produces higher weight and fluid loss compared with treatment with intravenous diuretics. In addition, UF also reduces a 90-day resource utilization in patients with ADHF. UF may thus prove to be an effective alternative to high doses of diuretic therapy in patients with ADHF, particularly in the presence of renal insufficiency.

Another small study designed for patients with ADHF investigated the effects of UF and standard intravenous diuretic (furosemide) therapy on the GFR and renal plasma flow [63]. The study comprised 19 patients who were randomized to receive UF ($n = 9$) or intravenous diuretics ($n = 10$). After treatment, no significant difference was seen in the GFR, renal plasma flow, and filtration fraction in the two groups. The difference in the net 48-h fluid removal between the two groups was also found to be insignificant. However, urine output during the first 48 h was significantly higher in the furosemide group than in the UF group.

The results of these randomized trials demonstrate that UF is associated with no major safety concerns, and compared with diuretics, it improves total fluid volume removal with decreased hospitalizations for CHF at 90 days in selected patients. However, the clinical trials have not evaluated theoretical concerns such as predisposition to infections and bleeding complications, which can be caused by the systemic heparinization and large-bore intravenous access needed during the UF procedure.

7. Systematic reviews and meta-analyses on HDF

Recently, several meta-analyses have been performed to compare UF with diuretics for treating volume overload in patients with ADHF. The first meta-analysis comprised nine studies involving 613 patients [22]. The mean weight loss in patients receiving UF therapy was 1.78 kg (95% CI −2.65 to −0.91 kg, $p < 0.001$). This loss was more than for those treated with standard diuretic therapy. However, between the two groups, there was little difference in post-intervention creatinine levels (mean change = −0.25 mg/dL, 95% CI −0.56 to 0.06 mg/dL, p = 0.112). In addition, the results showed that, compared with patients treated with standard diuretics, in those treated with UF, the risk of all-cause mortality persisted (pooled risk ratio = 1.00, 95% CI 0.64–1.56, p = 0.993).

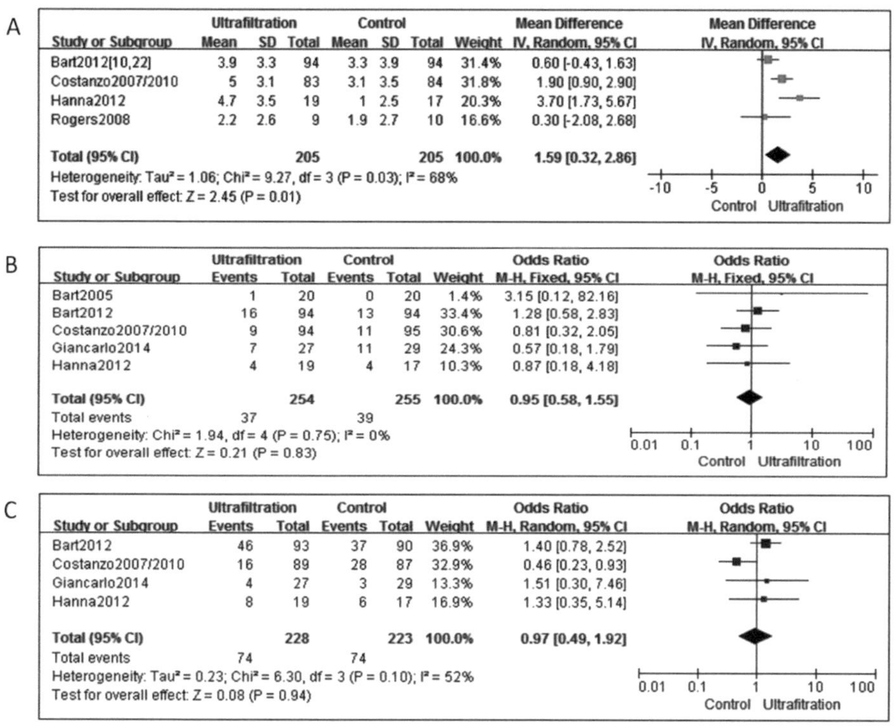

Figure 2. Forest plot of: a) Changes in weight loss at 48 h post therapy, b) all-cause mortality, c) all-cause rehospitalization. Reprinted from Cheng et al. [21], copyright with permission from International Heart Journal.

The second meta-analysis comprised seven RCTs with a total of 569 participants who met the eligibility criteria [21]. This analysis demonstrated that after 48 h of treatment, significantly higher amounts of weight loss and fluid removal were observed in the UF group compared with the diuretic group. Serum creatinine levels and changes in creatinine were found to be similar. There was no difference in all-cause mortality and all-cause rehospitalizations. In addition to these results, the authors noted that there were only minor differences between the UF and control groups in the incidence of adverse events, such as infections, anemia, hemorrhage, progressive HF, and other cardiac disorders (**Figure 2**).

8. Recommendations for the use of HDF in clinical practice

UF recommendations for HF from the 2013 guideline by the American College of Cardiology Foundation/American Heart Association Task Force [64] are shown in **Table 1**, along with recommendations from the Canadian Cardiovascular Society [65] and the European Society of Cardiology [66].

Reference	Guidelines
American College of Cardiology/ American Heart Association (2013)[64]	"Ultrafiltration may be considered for patients with obvious volume overload to alleviate congestive symptoms and fluid weight. Ultrafiltration may be considered for patients with refractory congestion not responding to medical therapy."
Canadian Cardiovascular Society (2012)[65]	"Venovenous ultrafiltration may be of benefit in relieving congestion particularly in diuretic-resistant patients"
European Society of Cardiology (2012)[66]	"Venovenous isolated ultrafiltration is sometimes used to remove fluid in patients with heart failure, although it is usually reserved for those unresponsive or resistant to diuretics."

Table 1. Recommendations and guidelines for the use of hemodiafiltration in patients with congestive heart failure.

9. HDF challenges and cost-effectiveness

Controversy still exists regarding the efficacy of HDF reported in clinical trial results to restore diuretic responsiveness in patients with CHF. The studies evaluating HDF showed considerable heterogeneity in terms of (1) study population, (2) causes of acute decompensation, (3) indications and protocols used for the prescription of HDF, (4) the "standard management" used in the control arm, and (5) end points. Marenzi et al. recommended using HDF as a complementary intervention along with diuretics rather than solely as an alternative intervention in patients with ADHF [52]. Moreover, HDF should probably be prescribed on an individual basis in diuretic-resistant patients to achieve safe decongestion. From a financial

http://dx.doi.org/10.5772/63393

standpoint, expenditures associated with HDF usage are still a major concern. Although initially these expenditures were considered non-prohibitive, a decision-model analysis has since found HDF to be expensive from a societal and hospital perspective. Nonetheless, for a Medicare payer, HDF can be cost-effective if existing nephrology resources such as dialysis machines, disposable supplies, and nursing staff are used as alternatives [67].

10. Conclusion

In patients with ADHF, decongestion is a major treatment goal. HDF techniques seem to be an effective tool for removal of fluid, but more robust studies are required to clarify the benefits of HDF and to characterize the group of patients who would benefit most from using it over standard diuretic therapy. Despite recent studies, crucial clinical questions are left unanswered. It is nonetheless apparent that HDF is an effective treatment strategy that should be used only for a selected group of suitable patients and performed by skilled professionals. The next research step for UF should not involve evaluating its effectiveness over that of diuretics; rather, it is more important to identify the patients who best respond to this technique to help restore their diuretic responsiveness.

Author details

Luai Alhazmi[1], Abdulelah Nuqali[2], Ankush Moza[2] and Mujeeb Sheikh[2*]

*Address all correspondence to: Mujeeb.sheikh@utoledo.edu

1 Department of Internal Medicine, University of Toledo Medical Center, Toledo, Ohio, USA

2 Division of Cardiovascular Medicine, Department of Internal Medicine, University of Toledo Medical Center, Toledo, Ohio, USA

References

[1] Hobbs F, Kenkre J, Roalfe A, et al. Impact of heart failure and left ventricular systolic dysfunction on quality of life. A cross-sectional study comparing common chronic cardiac and medical disorders and a representative adult population. European Heart Journal. 2002;23(23):1867–876.

[2] Bekelman DB, Havranek EP, Becker DM, et al. Symptoms, depression, and quality of life in patients with heart failure. Journal of Cardiac Failure. 2007;13(8):643–648.

[3] Klocek M, Czarnecka D. Quality of life in patients with chronic heart failure. In: Kalina Kawecka-Jaszcz, Marek Klocek, Beata Tobiasz-Adamczyk, Christopher J. Bulpitt Health-related quality of life in cardiovascular patients: Italy: Springer; 2013:61–73.

[4] Juenger J, Schellberg D, Kraemer S, et al. Health related quality of life in patients with congestive heart failure: comparison with other chronic diseases and relation to functional variables. Heart. 2002;87(3):235–241.

[5] Jencks SF, Williams MV, Coleman EA. Rehospitalizations among patients in the medicare fee-for-service program. New England Journal of Medicine. 2009;360(14): 1418–1428.

[6] Cowie M, Kirby M. Heart failure: an overview. Managing heart failure in primary care: a practical guide. Oxfordshire, UK: Bladon Medical Publishing; 2001.

[7] Stewart S, MacIntyre K, Hole DJ, et al. More 'malignant' than cancer? Five-year survival following a first admission for heart failure. European Journal of Heart Failure. 2001;3(3):315–322.

[8] Mozaffarian D, Benjamin EJ, Go AS, et al. Heart disease and stroke statistics—2016 update. A report from the American Heart Association. Circulation. 2015:CIR. 0000000000000350.

[9] Adams KF, Fonarow GC, Emerman CL, et al. Characteristics and outcomes of patients hospitalized for heart failure in the United States: rationale, design, and preliminary observations from the first 100,000 cases in the Acute Decompensated Heart Failure National Registry (ADHERE). American Heart Journal. 2005;149(2):209–216.

[10] Chen H-Y, Chou K-J, Fang H-C, et al. Effect of ultrafiltration versus intravenous furosemide for decompensated heart failure in cardiorenal syndrome: a systematic review with meta-analysis of randomized controlled trials. Nephron. 2015;129(3):189–196.

[11] Metra M, Cleland JG, Weatherley BD, et al. Dyspnoea in patients with acute heart failure: an analysis of its clinical course, determinants, and relationship to 60-day outcomes in the PROTECT pilot study. European Journal of Heart Failure. 2010;12(5): 499–507.

[12] Metra M, Teerlink JR, Felker GM, et al. Dyspnoea and worsening heart failure in patients with acute heart failure: results from the Pre-RELAX-AHF study. European Journal of Heart Failure. 2010;12(10):1130–1139.

[13] Gheorghiade M, Filippatos G. Reassessing treatment of acute heart failure syndromes: the ADHERE registry. European Heart Journal Supplements. 2005;7(suppl B):B13–B19.

[14] Domanski M, Norman J, Pitt B, et al. Diuretic use, progressive heart failure, and death in patients in the studies of left ventricular dysfunction (SOLVD). Journal of the American College of Cardiology. 2003;42(4):705–708.

[15] Kittleson M, Hurwitz S, Shah MR, et al. Development of circulatory-renal limitations to angiotensin-converting enzyme inhibitors identifies patients with severe heart failure and early mortality. Journal of the American College of Cardiology. 2003;41(11): 2029–2035.

[16] Felker GM, Lee KL, Bull DA, et al. Diuretic strategies in patients with acute decompensated heart failure. New England Journal of Medicine. 2011;364(9):797–805.

[17] Guazzi MD, Agostoni P, Perego B, et al. Apparent paradox of neurohumoral axis inhibition after body fluid volume depletion in patients with chronic congestive heart failure and water retention. British Heart Journal. 1994;72(6):534–539.

[18] Marenzi G, Lauri G, Grazi M, et al. Circulatory response to fluid overload removal by extracorporeal ultrafiltration in refractory congestive heart failure. Journal of the American College of Cardiology. 2001;38(4):963–968.

[19] Kwong JS, Yu C-M. Ultrafiltration for acute decompensated heart failure: a systematic review and meta-analysis of randomized controlled trials. International Journal of Cardiology. 2014;172(2):395–402.

[20] Zhi Q, Liang JC. Diuretics and ultrafiltration in acute heart failure syndrom. International Heart Journal. 2013;54(6):390–394.

[21] Cheng Z, Wang L, Gu Y, et al. Efficacy and safety of ultrafiltration in decompensated heart failure patients with renal insufficiency. International Heart Journal. 2015;56(3): 319–323.

[22] Ebrahim B, Sindhura K, Okoroh J, et al. Meta-analysis of ultrafiltration versus diuretics treatment option for overload volume reduction in patients with acute decompensated heart failure. Arquivos Brasileiros de Cardiologia. 2015;104(5):417–425.

[23] Verbrugge FH, Mullens W, Tang WW. Management of cardio-renal syndrome and diuretic resistance. Current Treatment Options in Cardiovascular Medicine. 2016;18(2): 1–15.

[24] Testani JM, Brisco MA, Turner JM, et al. Loop diuretic efficiency: a metric of diuretic responsiveness with prognostic importance in acute decompensated heart failure. Circulation: Heart Failure. 2013;DOI: CIRCHEARTFAILURE. 113.000895.

[25] Valente MA, Voors AA, Damman K, et al. Diuretic response in acute heart failure: clinical characteristics and prognostic significance. European Heart Journal. 2014;35(19):1284–1293.

[26] Singh D, Shrestha K, Testani JM, et al. Insufficient natriuretic response to continuous intravenous furosemide is associated with poor long-term outcomes in acute decompensated heart failure. Journal of Cardiac Failure. 2014;20(6):392–399.

[27] Aronson D, Burger AJ. Diuretic response: clinical and hemodynamic predictors and relation to clinical outcome. Journal of Cardiac Failure, 22 (3), pp. 193–200.

[28] Ter Maaten JM, Dunning AM, Valente MA, et al. Diuretic response in acute heart failure —an analysis from ASCEND-HF. American Heart Journal. 2015;170(2):313–321. e314.

[29] Verbrugge F, Dupont M, Bertrand P, et al. Determinants and impact of the natriuretic response to diuretic therapy in heart failure with reduced ejection fraction and volume overload. ACTA CARDIOLOGICA, 2015, 70 (3), p. 265-273.

[30] Kumar D, Bagarhatta R. Fractional excretion of sodium and its association with prognosis of decompensated heart failure patients. Journal of Clinical and Diagnostic Research: JCDR. 2015;9(4):OC01.

[31] Voors AA, Davison BA, Teerlink JR, et al. Diuretic response in patients with acute decompensated heart failure: characteristics and clinical outcome—an analysis from RELAX-AHF. European Journal of Heart Failure. 2014;16(11):1230–1240.

[32] http://www.nhlbi.nih.gov/meetings/workshops/cardiorenal-hf-hd.htm. Accessed February 2, 2016.

[33] Ronco C, Haapio M, House AA, et al. Cardiorenal syndrome. Journal of the American College of Cardiology. 2008;52(19):1527–1539.

[34] Ronco C, Cicoira M, McCullough PA. Cardiorenal syndrome type 1: pathophysiological crosstalk leading to combined heart and kidney dysfunction in the setting of acutely decompensated heart failure. Journal of the American College of Cardiology. 2012;60(12):1031–1042.

[35] Hunt SA, Abraham WT, Chin MH, et al. 2009 focused update incorporated into the ACC/AHA 2005 guidelines for the diagnosis and management of heart failure in adults: a report of the American College of Cardiology Foundation/American Heart Association Task Force on Practice Guidelines developed in collaboration with the International Society for Heart and Lung Transplantation. Journal of the American College of Cardiology. 2009;53(15):e1–e90.

[36] Metra M, Davison B, Bettari L, et al. Is worsening renal function an ominous prognostic sign in patients with acute heart failure? The role of congestion and its interaction with renal function. Circulation: Heart Failure. 2011:CIRCHEARTFAILURE. 111.963413.

[37] Bart BA, Goldsmith SR, Lee KL, et al. Ultrafiltration in decompensated heart failure with cardiorenal syndrome. New England Journal of Medicine. 2012;367(24):2296–2304.

[38] Freda BJ, Slawsky M, Mallidi J, et al. Decongestive treatment of acute decompensated heart failure: cardiorenal implications of ultrafiltration and diuretics. American Journal of Kidney Diseases. 2011;58(6):1005–1017.

[39] Bock JS, Gottlieb SS. Cardiorenal syndrome: new perspectives. Circulation. 2010;121(23):2592–2600.

[40] Shamseddin MK, Parfrey PS. Mechanisms of the cardiorenal syndromes. Nature Reviews Nephrology. 2009;5(11):641–649.

[41] Fröhlich H, Katus HA, Täger T, et al. Peritoneal ultrafiltration in end-stage chronic heart failure. Clinical Kidney Journal. 2015:sfv007.

[42] Bertoli SV, Musetti C, Ciurlino D, et al. Peritoneal ultrafiltration in refractory heart failure: a cohort study. Peritoneal Dialysis International. 2014;34(1):64–70.

[43] Lu R, Muciño-Bermejo M-J, Ribeiro LC, et al. Peritoneal dialysis in patients with refractory congestive heart failure: a systematic review. Cardiorenal Medicine. 2015;5(2):145–156.

[44] Marshall MR, Creamer JM, Foster M, et al. Mortality rate comparison after switching from continuous to prolonged intermittent renal replacement for acute kidney injury in three intensive care units from different countries. Nephrology Dialysis Transplantation. 2011;26(7):2169–2175.

[45] Schwenger V, Weigand MA, Hoffmann O, et al. Sustained low efficiency dialysis using a single-pass batch system in acute kidney injury-a randomized interventional trial: the Renal Replacement Therapy Study in Intensive Care Unit Patients. Critical Care. 2012;16(4):R140.

[46] Kron J, Kron S, Wenkel R, et al. Extended daily on-line high-volume haemodiafiltration in septic multiple organ failure: a well-tolerated and feasible procedure. Nephrology Dialysis Transplantation. 2012;27(1):146–152.

[47] Fieghen HE, Friedrich JO, Burns KE, et al. The hemodynamic tolerability and feasibility of sustained low efficiency dialysis in the management of critically ill patients with acute kidney injury. BMC Nephrology. 2010;11(1):1.

[48] Tolwani A. Continuous renal-replacement therapy for acute kidney injury. New England Journal of Medicine. 2012;367(26):2505–2514.

[49] Iorio L, Violi F, Simonelli R, et al. [Sustained low-efficiency dialysis (SLED) in patients with prevalent systolic heart failure refractory to medical treatment and with chronic renal failure]. Giornale italiano di nefrologia: organo ufficiale della Societa italiana di nefrologia. 2006;23 Suppl 34:S71–73.

[50] Violi F, Nacca RG, Iengo G, et al. [Long-term sustained low efficiency dialysis in eight patients with class IV NYHA heart failure resistant to high-dose diuretic treatment]. Giornale italiano di nefrologia: organo ufficiale della Societa italiana di nefrologia. 2009;26 Suppl 46:50–52.

[51] Fleming GM. Renal replacement therapy review: past, present and future. Organogenesis. 2011;7(1):2–12.

[52] Marenzi G, Morpurgo M, Agostoni P. Continuous ultrafiltration in acute decompensated heart failure: current issues and future directions. American Journal of Cardiovascular Drugs. 2015;15(2):103–112.

[53] Silverstein M, Ford C, Lysaght M, et al. Treatment of severe fluid overload by ultrafiltration. Survey of Anesthesiology. 1975;19(6):521–522.

[54] Canaud B, Leblanc M, Leray-Moragues H, et al. Slow continuous and daily ultrafiltration for refractory congestive heart failure. Nephrology Dialysis Transplantation. 1998;13(90004):51–55.

[55] Giglioli C, Landi D, Cecchi E, et al. Effects of ULTRAfiltration vs. DIureticS on clinical, biohumoral and haemodynamic variables in patients with deCOmpensated heart failure: the ULTRADISCO study. European Journal of Heart Failure. 2011;13(3):337–346.

[56] Agostoni P, Marenzi G, Lauri G, et al. Sustained improvement in functional capacity after removal of body fluid with isolated ultrafiltration in chronic cardiac insufficiency: failure of furosemide to provide the same result. The American Journal of Medicine. 1994;96(3):191–199.

[57] Rimondini A, Cipolla CM, Della Bella P, et al. Hemofiltration as short-term treatment for refractory congestive heart failure. The American Journal of Medicine. 1987;83(1): 43–48.

[58] Radzishevsky E, Salman N, Paz H, et al. First experience in ambulatory ultrafiltration therapy for congested heart failure patients in Israel: a feasibility study. The Israel Medical Association Journal: IMAJ. 2015;17(1):24–26.

[59] Teo L, Lim C, Neo C, et al. Ultrafiltration in patients with decompensated heart failure and diuretic resistance: an Asian centre experience. Giornale italiano di nefrologia: organo ufficiale della Societa italiana di nefrologia, 2005, 23: S71-3.

[60] Costanzo MR, Negoianu D, Jaski BE, et al. Aquapheresis versus intravenous diuretics and hospitalizations for heart failure. Journal of Cardiac Failure, 2015, 21.11: 937-939.

[61] Bart BA, Boyle A, Bank AJ, et al. Ultrafiltration versus usual care for hospitalized patients with heart failure: the Relief for Acutely Fluid-Overloaded Patients With Decompensated Congestive Heart Failure (RAPID-CHF) trial. Journal of the American College of Cardiology. 2005;46(11):2043–2046.

[62] Costanzo MR, Guglin ME, Saltzberg MT, et al. Ultrafiltration versus intravenous diuretics for patients hospitalized for acute decompensated heart failure. Journal of the American College of Cardiology. 2007;49(6):675–683.

[63] Rogers HL, Marshall J, Bock J, et al. A randomized, controlled trial of the renal effects of ultrafiltration as compared to furosemide in patients with acute decompensated heart failure. Journal of Cardiac Failure. 2008;14(1):1–5.

[64] Yancy CW, Jessup M, Bozkurt B, et al. 2013 ACCF/AHA guideline for the management of heart failure: a report of the American College of Cardiology Foundation/American Heart Association Task Force on Practice Guidelines. Journal of the American College of Cardiology. 2013;62(16):e147–e239.

[65] McKelvie RS, Moe GW, Ezekowitz JA, et al. The 2012 Canadian Cardiovascular Society heart failure management guidelines update: focus on acute and chronic heart failure. Canadian Journal of Cardiology. 2013;29(2):168–181.

[66] McMurray JJ, Adamopoulos S, Anker SD, et al. ESC Guidelines for the diagnosis and treatment of acute and chronic heart failure 2012. European Journal of Heart Failure. 2012;14(8):803–869.

[67] Kazory A. Ultrafiltration therapy for heart failure: trials and tribulations. Clinical Journal of the American Society of Nephrology. 2013:CJN. 02910313.

Chapter 6

Update on Clinical Evidence Supporting Hemodiafiltration

Bernard Canaud, Aileen Grassmann,
Laura Scatizzi and Daniele Marcelli

Additional information is available at the end of the chapter

http://dx.doi.org/10.5772/63027

Abstract

The aim of this chapter is to define hemodiafiltration target efficiency, to clarify the concept of "optimal convective dose," and to facilitate hemodiafiltration (HDF) implementation in clinical practice by addressing the need for the establishment of best clinical practices for HDF. The approach taken was to conduct a comprehensive summary of clinical evidence supporting HDF. Convective dose is the total ultrafiltered volume and is complementary to diffusive dose (urea Kt/V) as a dose-dependent parameter. It can be quantified and adjusted to patient characteristics. Factors affecting convective dose are discussed: patient characteristics, prescription-dependent factors, and technical and machine-dependent factors. The key issue of HDF prescription and implementation of best practices is addressed as are intermediary and endpoint clinical outcomes. The main messages are as follows: (1) HDF is safe and effective provided that best clinical practices are followed and the right convective dose is delivered; (2) HDF is easy to perform with new technology; and (3) depending on the convection volume, HDF reduces all-cause and cardiovascular mortality. Open challenges remain, namely, the implementation of best practices to (a) achieve optimal convection volume, (b) define patient subsets that would benefit more from HDF, and (c) evaluate new tools that fine-tune HDF prescription according to individual patient needs.

Keywords: convective dose, substitution modality, treatment outcome, convection volume, clinical evidence

1. Introduction

Conventional diffusion-based dialysis modalities, namely, low-flux and even high-flux hemodialysis (HD), are limited in their capacity to effectively remove large uremic toxins and to improve outcomes for chronic kidney disease (CKD) patients [1]. By increasing convective solute transport, hemodiafiltration (HDF) enhances solute removal capacity over a broad range of middle- and large-size uremic toxins implicated in the pathophysiology of CKD [2, 3]. In addition, convective-based modalities have been shown to improve hemodynamic stability [4, 5] and to reduce patients' inflammation profile—both factors implicated in CKD morbidity and mortality [6–8]. Growing clinical evidence indicates that HDF-based modalities provide CKD patients with a number of clinical and biological benefits, including improved outcomes. Interestingly, it has recently emerged that the clinical benefits associated with HDF are positively associated with the total volume of fluid removed by ultrafiltration per session or per week [9–12]. This finding adds a new component to the conventional dialysis adequacy concept, namely, convective dose.

In this chapter, we elucidate the concept of convective dose and discuss the threshold above which an improvement in CKD patient outcome can be expected. In addition, factors implicated in the achievement of an optimal convective dose in the sense of best clinical practice are reviewed and clinical evidence supporting the use of HDF today is summarized.

1.1. Why is hemodiafiltration needed?

From a nephrologist's perspective, it is disappointing to observe that outcomes of end-stage kidney disease (ESKD) patients remain poor despite significant progress in hemodialyzer performances, HD machines and monitoring devices, better understanding of uremic toxicity, and improved patient management. Even without an in-depth analysis of root causes and reasons for renal replacement therapy (RRT) limitations, several factors are easily recognizable as contributing to this outcome. It is usually convenient to group these into two categories: "nonmodifiable factors," such as age, gender, ethnicity, comorbidity profile, and kidney disease history, and "modifiable factors," such as RRT modality and treatment adequacy. Changing the renal replacement treatment paradigm and improving practice patterns to ensure customized and better care are the only ways to improve the outcomes of ESKD patients.

In this context, two main options are available. First, HDF is today's most innovative, promising, and advanced alternative to high-flux HD. By combining diffusive and enhanced convective solute mass transfer, HDF offers the most efficient RRT today over a wide spectrum of uremic toxins including middle- and large-sized solutes. Using ultrapure dialysis fluids (water and dialysis fluid), HDF constitutes a highly biocompatible system and suppresses the occurrence of microinflammation processes [13–15]. By reducing the incidence of hypotensive episodes as well as dialysis intolerance symptoms [16–18], HDF may reduce or prevent repetitive cardiovascular insults and their deleterious long-term consequences. By giving access to an unlimited amount of substitution fluid at the cost of ultrapure dialysis fluid, online HDF provides a cost-effective approach for optimizing and customizing HDF treatment prescription to the patient's metabolic needs. Provided that best clinical practices and hygienic rules are applied, HDF offers a reliable, efficient, and cost-effective RRT tool.

Second, the extension of treatment time is the more physiologic approach to improving patient outcome, even if not the most popular one. Increasing treatment time and/or frequency is the best way to facilitate sodium mass removal and thereby restore extracellular fluid volume, to ensure removal of uremic compounds with low intracorporeal mass transfer coefficients or tightly bound to albumin, and to minimize "nonphysiological" changes due to the aggressive nature of intermittent treatment schedules. These two approaches, HDF and extended treatment time, should not be considered competitive but rather complementary. Only a few studies have combined the solute mass transfer capacity of HDF with increased treatment time [19–21] and all clinical trials have confirmed the tremendous benefits of such combination on intermediary and long-term outcomes.

1.2. What is the clinical evidence for hemodiafiltration?

Although many studies associate HDF with significant improvements in ESKD patient outcomes, still some conflicting data or cost concerns have hampered general clinical and widespread acceptance of this method. Here, we attempt to reconcile facts and concerns regarding HDF. To begin, it should be stressed that a differentiated understanding of HDF should be adopted as opposed to considering HDF to be a generic term that covers all convection-based renal replacement modalities. The differentiation necessary lies in the magnitude of the convection dose that must be delivered to improve outcomes of ESKD patients. Based on published literature and our own experience, we revisit the current definition of convective dose and its threshold value for improved patient outcome, we review the factors affecting convective dose delivery, we summarize the best clinical practices in HDF prescription, and we summarize the main studies addressing clinical outcomes.

2. Convective dose concept—from minimal to optimal dosage

According to the EUDIAL group recommendations, convective dose is the total volume of ultrafiltration achieved per HDF session (L/session) and summed to week (L/week), standardized to postdilution convection volume for the various other dilution modalities (i.e., pre-, mixed, or mid-HDF), taking differences in the fluid volumes into consideration [22]. This is an easy and clinically relevant surrogate indicator of the convective component. Knowing that only hemodialyzers containing membranes that are highly permeable to both water (Kuf>50) and solutes (sieving coefficient β2-microglobulin [β2M] >0.6) are used for HDF, it is possible to calculate the convective component of solute clearance. An alternative proposal was to focus more on the biological effect of middle-molecule removal using biomarkers that reflect the convective action of the HDF. Among uremic toxins, β2M, a 12-kDa peptide, seems to be the most clinically relevant representative of the middle-molecule uremic toxins and strongly implicated in both morbidity and mortality of CKD patients.

Following international guidelines, urea Kt/V has been established as the principle dialysis dose quantifier and is regularly used as a quality-control tool for treatment delivery. To be valid, this approach requires certified methodology (appropriate urea sampling method and time, suitable formula) and appropriate timing of measurements (minimum of once monthly) to capture early deviation in dialysis efficacy. The ionic dialysance (iK) measurement embedded in some HD monitors is an option. This offers an interesting and cost-effective alternative that may be performed routinely at each session providing a true continuous quality-control tool. Using then the simplified concept of iKt, where iK stands for the average ionic dialysance measured by HD monitor and t stands for the duration of the dialysis session, one can estimate the total diffusive dose delivered per session (L/session).

The effective total dialysis dose (i.e., diffusive and convective) delivered to the ESKD patient can be easily assessed. Convective dose as estimated by total ultrafiltered volume per session (L/session) could be considered as a complementary component of the diffusive dose delivered and estimated by iKt (L/session).

A systematic review of studies [retrospective cohorts, prospective randomized controlled trial (RCT)] exploring the relationship of convective dose and patient outcome has shown that survival benefit is observed only when a minimum threshold ultrafiltration volume has been delivered [23]. The critical ultrafiltration volume per session (or per week) required for better patient outcome is between 20 and 22 L/session for a typical European ESKD patient. More recently, it has been shown that total ultrafiltered volume per session (or per week) acted as a continuous variable mimicking a sigmoidal dose-response curve [24].

The normalization of the convective dose to the patient's anthropometric characteristics has been proposed to match with patient metabolic needs and also to facilitate the generalization of this relationship with different patient profiles (e.g., Asian and American). In fact, such normalization attempts using different scalings (i.e., body weight, height, body surface area, and total body water) have been adopted in different studies, including the Estudio de Supervivencia de Hemodiafiltración On-Line (ESHOL) [25] and the individual personal data meta-analysis that was part of the European pooled project [26]. Interestingly, none of these scaling factors have enhanced sensitivity in predicting the relative risk (RR) of mortality. Crude convection volume per session (or per week) or convection volume scaled to body surface area or total body water tend to perform best in predicting survival benefits or mortality risks where HDF is concerned.

3. Factors affecting convective dose

Best clinical practices are essential in daily practice to achieve optimal ultrafiltration flow and the total ultrafiltered volume targeted. Schematically, three basic components need to be considered: patient-dependent factors, prescription-dependent factors, and technical or machine-dependent factors.

3.1. Patient-dependent factors

3.1.1. Vascular access

The achievement of "high" blood flows (>350 mL/min) depends on the type of vascular access (i.e., central venous catheter, arteriovenous fistula, or graft) and on the provision and maintenance of vascular access patency. Vascular access is defined as inadequate when an extracorporeal blood flow of at least 300 mL/min cannot be reached. Basically, patients treated with online HDF require a vascular access capable of delivering a consistent extracorporeal blood flow between 350 and 400 mL/min or higher. Such extracorporeal blood flows could be reached with large bore tunneled central venous catheters and with arteriovenous fistulas or grafts delivering access flows of ≥500 mL/min. High blood flow is essential to ensure that a sufficient amount of blood is processed during the treatment session. Vascular access flow performances and needle sizes assume a fundamental role in preserving the advantages of applying a high convection volume.

3.1.2. Individual patient criteria

Hematocrit and protocrit (the volume fraction of plasma proteins that may be calculated as the product of 0.000718 and the total protein concentration of plasma proteins in g/mL [22]) affect negatively the plasma water volume and plasma water flow. High hematocrit (e.g., resulting from anemia management and hemoglobin targets) and high total protein concentration (e.g., due to the particular nutritional and inflammatory status of the patient) enhance viscosity tremendously, reduce ultrafiltration capacity (filtration fraction), and provide unfavorable conditions for ultrafiltration flow. The additional ultrafiltration applied to achieve a given weight loss is an additive factor that may affect total ultrafiltration. Finally, a dynamic interaction between blood flow (shear rate and shear stress), blood components (hematocrit and protocrit), filtration fraction (ultrafiltration flow to blood flow ratio), and membrane surface (protein layer formation) is crucial to facilitate ultrafiltration flow. Many of these factors are taken into consideration in modern dialysis machine technology.

3.2. Prescription-dependent factors

3.2.1. Blood flow

The effective extracorporeal blood flow delivered is a fundamental determinant of all extracorporeal cleansing therapies. Among factors that determine the efficiency with which uremic solutes are removed during dialysis, extracorporeal blood flow, whether instantaneous (flow rate) or cumulative (total blood volume processed over the session), is the most critical. Treatment efficiency assessed either in terms of solute clearance or solute mass removal is then dependent on the total blood "processed" within a dialysis session.

High blood flows are critical in HDF, as they have a dual action, one being to maximize the amount of solute removed and the other being to preserve membrane permeability by retarding the formation of a protein layer on the membrane (secondary layer formation). The choice of needle size matters in HDF. Following Poiseuille's law, needle size is a barrier to high blood flow: 15-gauge needles (optimally 14-gauge needles) are required to sustain blood flow of ≥350 mL/min at an acceptable pressure regimen.

3.2.2. Choice of hemodiafilter

The choice of a specifically designed hemodiafilter is important to optimize ultrafiltration flow and prevent dysfunction or alarms occurring on the HDF monitor due to hemorheological changes in the dialyzer. Preferred hemodiafilter features, apart from being equipped with highly permeable membranes, should favor the following to reduce internal convective processes: low blood flow resistance (large lumen diameter of fibers (e.g., 200 μm), short length of dialyzer housing, and increased number of fibers per sectional surface area.

3.2.3. Anticoagulation

Methods of anticoagulation will not addressed here in detail. However, anticoagulation is required to prevent thrombosis of extracorporeal blood circuit and to ensure a safe and efficient HDF session. Different kinds of antithrombotic agents can be used systematically by intravenous (IV) injection.

Unfractionated heparin (UH) is administered as an IV bolus dose (30–50 IU/kg) at the start of the HDF session followed by continuous IV infusion (500–700 IU/h). The heparin dosing regimen for HDF does not differ from that in regular HD.

The use of low molecular weight heparin (LMWH) is nowadays favored by many centers because of its ease of use and its better risk profile. In this case, LMWH should be preferably administered IV into the venous line and not into the arterial line to prevent significant loss during the first hemodialyzer passage.

3.2.4. Treatment time prescription

The prescription of HDF treatment time duration and frequency is usually based on the patient's metabolic needs, extracellular fluid management, and cardiovascular and session tolerance. Increasing both the duration and frequency will facilitate the delivery of a high volume of ultrafiltration. A pragmatic approach is to establish a suitable convective dose for a given patient and to increase the treatment time according to the limitation of effective blood flow delivery.

3.3. Technical or machine-dependent factors

3.3.1. Transmembrane pressure management

Achieving high ultrafiltration rates and targeted ultrafiltration volumes can be challenging and requires the careful management of the transmembrane pressure (TMP) according to the treatment modality selected. In attempting to achieve high ultrafiltration volumes, hemoconcentration within the filter commonly results in high TMP, triggering pressure alarms and potentially causing cell damage. Basically, the augmented protein layer formation occurring naturally at the blood-membrane surface during the course of the HDF session fouls the membrane pores and reduces the membrane's hydraulic permeability. In combination with the increased oncotic pressure (total protein increase) along the fibers, this tends to reduce the ultrafiltration flow. Faced with situations of high TMP increase and/or pressure alarms, nursing staff manually reduce the substitution flow and thus reduce the chances of achieving the targeted ultrafiltration volume.

3.3.2. Machine options

New features to optimize HDF performances and achieve optimal convective doses are currently available. The adjustment of the substitution mode was the most obvious and primary focus of investigation. When postdilution is problematic, switching to pre-, mixed, or mid-dilution mode may be a viable alternative. In all these cases, the targeted convection volume needs to be adjusted for the dilution factor corresponding to the HDF modality chosen (e.g., x2 for predilution HDF or x1.5 for mid-dilution HDF in manual prescription) to match efficacy with the postdilution mode.

New technical features involving specific software algorithms are currently being implemented and tested in new online HDF machines. Basically, the idea is to provide an automatic ultrafiltration control system to reduce membrane fouling and ensure maximal ultrafiltration flow considering basic operational conditions of blood flow, hemorheological conditions, and prescription setting. Schematically, the system avoids excessive hemoconcentration by the continuous adaptation of the substitution flow according to changes in blood viscosity within the dialyzer as identified by signal analyses of the pressure pulses transmitted from the peristaltic blood pump. Signal analysis is conducted several times per minute, and the substitution rate is automatically adapted based on pressure pulse attenuation and cross-membrane pressure assessment. Using such automatic control systems, it is possible to increase the ultrafiltered volume per session by 10 to 20% without harming the patient, filter, or cells.

3.3.3. Other machine-related variables

As mentioned previously, treatment time is one of the factors limiting the increase of "dialysis dose". In the current models of delivering dialysis in dialysis units, based on shifts assigned to nurses with a ratio of one nurse to three to five patients, any further increase of treatment time has an associated cost. Out of the 5.5 to 6 h of the shift length for each single nurse, it is possible to deliver a median of 4 h of treatment to three to five patients. There are two ways to achieve a cost-neutral increase in treatment time. The first is to reduce the time needed to prepare the dialysis equipment before initiating treatment. Faster disinfection of the dialysis machine is achievable with more simple hydraulic components and/or more effective disinfection processes. Also, the disinfection of the machine surface can be simpler, safer, and faster; this is achievable with especially designed equipment surfaces having as few discontinuities as possible. The second way is to reduce the number and complexity of nurse interventions. This approach may allow nurses to treat more patients, thus decreasing the cost of treatment for each patient per hour. Consequently, it could be possible to increase the time of the shift and the treatment time in a cost-neutral manner. Is this possible? According to Tsobanelis et al. [27], new dialysis equipment under testing in HDF mode for fistula patients had a 24% reduction in the number of major handling steps compared to the previous dialysis machine from the same company.

Other aspects to be considered when targeting an increase of patient to nurse ratio are those related to safety. The risk of harm has to be reduced as much as possible, and one option is to reduce this risk by the improved design of the equipment. As an example, we can again mention the recent experience of Tsobanelis et al. [28], who reported that the tested new equipment had 27% fewer major process steps and touch points critical to hygiene compared to the current machine version. The authors found it particularly noteworthy that it was possible to avoid disconnection of the arterial line from the arterial needle with the redesigned process of blood reinfusion at the end of the session.

Finally, in the time of green economy, the authors also highlighted that the switch from an infusion line to an integrated infusion port reduced the volume of contaminated waste. The major source of waste relates to the disposables (bloodlines and dialyzers), so that newly designed, integrated disposables can facilitate a reduction of disposable waste, for example, of approximately 0.2 kg/session as reported by Schleser et al. [29], which, given an average of 10,000 treatments yearly delivered by a dialysis unit, translates into 2000 kg less waste. In terms of carbon footprint, one should also consider the consumption of water and energy and how this can be limited, for example, by having a more efficient water treatment system.

4. HDF prescription and implementation of best practices

4.1. Current status

Online HDF can no longer be considered an experimental treatment but has now developed into a mature and accepted RRT. In fact, this dialysis modality is employed for sustaining the lives of more than 160,000 ESKD patients worldwide, including 80,000 in Europe, Middle East, and Africa. Europe played a leading role in developing this therapy, where the prevalence of HDF is close to 18% (varying across countries from 0 to 100%). The annual growth rate is approximately 6% [30]. In 2013, Japan treated 31,273 patients with HDF (23,445 thereof on online HDF), representing 10% of its total dialysis population (294,605 patients; Kawanishi, personal data). The number increased by 4% between 2013 and 2014 as positively influenced by the implementation of a specific reimbursement fee in 2012. Interestingly, in Japan, the predominant HDF mode is predilution HDF (90.8% of HDF treatments).

4.2. Treatment schedule prescription

The prescription of the HDF treatment schedule is based on the usual target of providing optimal RRT to the ESKD patient. It is a composite and trade-off between patient-specific issues (e.g., metabolic needs, treatment tolerance and acceptance, and patient-treatment interaction), local logistical and practical issues (e.g., facility and/or modality availability), and health regulation and reimbursement policies.

The duration and frequency of sessions are based on two main components: (1) patient's metabolic needs and dialysis adequacy targets and (2) extracellular fluid management and cardiovascular tolerance depending on ultrafiltration rate. Increasing session length and frequency will facilitate the achievement of a high ultrafiltration volume. A pragmatic approach is to estimate a suitable convective dose for a given patient and to increase the treatment time according to the limitations present regarding effective blood flow or other hemorheological factors.

In clinical practice, prescription comprises the setting of the substitution rate (substitution volume per session extended to weekly volume) and adding the required weight loss to achieve the dry weight for that patient. Based on the results of recent studies, a minimal substitution volume of 60 L/week (or 40 L/m^2 body surface area) is required in individual ESKD patients to improve patient outcome. The additional ultrafiltration volume required for the correction of extracellular fluid volume excess has to be added to the substitution volume.

The hemodialyzer used for HDF must contain membranes that are highly permeable for both water (Kuf>50 mL/h/mmHg) and solutes (sieving coefficient for $\beta 2M \geq 0.6$) with adequate dialyzer surface area. Filter design should favor a low internal blood flow resistance, thereby reducing membrane fouling and minimizing backfiltration as much as possible. A simple rule of thumb commonly applied in clinical practice is to consider 1 m^2/each 200 mL/min effective extracorporeal blood flow, meaning that a 2.0 m^2 hemodialyzer is appropriate for a blood flow of 400 mL/min [31].

In the past, the composition of the dialysis fluid differed from that of the substitution fluid. This is not the case in online HDF. Given the current definition of convective treatment adequacy, based on 23 L/session of convective dose in postdilution HDF, this equality of fluid compositions, and also the HDF mode, may affect the mass balance of electrolytes during the treatment session. Several studies dealing with the dialysate/substitution fluid prescription and focusing on sodium, calcium, and bicarbonate have been published.

Sodium: The importance of the correct sodium balancing during dialysis, preventing sodium overload with resultant thirst and water overload, has long been recognized. This risk of sodium loading also has to be considered in high efficiency treatments coupling diffusion and high volume convection. In a 1991 evaluation of HDF sessions with convective doses ranging between 9.1 and 16.7 L/week, Pedrini et al. [32] found that sodium balance was mainly affected by the sodium concentration gradient between initial plasma water and dialysate, the sodium level in the substitution fluid, and the imposed ultrafiltration rate. In the same patients treated with similar operating conditions, significantly lower net sodium removal was observed when on predilution compared to postdilution HDF [33]. Despite the complexity of managing the multifactorial equations describing the relationship between affecting variables and sodium balance (e.g., the laboratory method for the determination of sodium and the negative charge of plasma proteins) [33], ideal modern equipment should be able to automatically address sodium balance.

Calcium: The target in the case of calcium is to maintain a neutral calcium balance, as an excessive calcium load has been associated with vascular calcification, whereas calcium depletion has been linked to worsening secondary hyperparathyroidism and decreased bone mass [34]. Here also, the modality of HDF affects the balance. Although calcium balance during postdilution online HDF does not differ from standard HD, it is usually recommended to increase the dialysate/substitution fluid calcium concentration by 0.25 mmol/L in predilution HDF mode in order [34]. In addition, discrepancies between expected and observed concentrations in the dialysate/substitution fluid play an important role in the case of online HDF. In a volumetric system based on conductivity, the sodium for the bicarbonate dialysate/substitution fluid comes in part from a basic component and in part from an acidic component. In cases of a decrease in dialysate sodium with concomitant increase of bicarbonate, a lower proportion of the acid component will produce a lower than expected calcium level in the dialysate/substitution fluid [35].

Bicarbonate: a positive bicarbonate balance is targeted during the treatment session to neutralize the interdialytic accumulation of strong acid anions and to avoid starting the next session with metabolic acidosis. However, there is also a risk of postdialysis alkalosis. In a recent publication by Havlin et al. [36] analyzing 68 patients on postdilution HDF treated for 4 to 5 h with 80 to 90 mL/min of substitution fluid (19–27 L/session) with a dialysate bicarbonate concentration of 32 mmol/L, 34% of patients were acidotic at dialysis initiation, but 80% had metabolic alkalosis after dialysis. They speculated that this was due to an excessive elimination of retained and endogenous anions. According to the authors, this observation requires further investigation. In any case, several factors affect the mass balance. A significantly lower bicarbonate gain was observed in predilution HDF versus postdilution HDF [37]. As is true for all electrolytes, the difference in concentration between bicarbonate levels in the dialysate/substitution fluid and in the blood at the initiation of the session is positively correlated to the mass transfer. Therefore, to maintain the same bicarbonate balance when moving from postdilution HDF to predilution HDF, dialysate bicarbonate concentration should be increased by 2 mmol/L. In fact, in predilution HDF, bicarbonate levels of the blood entering in the dialyzer increase, enhancing the loss across the membrane and reducing the normal gain by diffusion from dialysis fluid to blood [33].

5. Clinical outcomes

5.1. Intermediary treatment outcomes (short-term studies)

In this section, intermediary treatment outcomes stand for surrogates of primary outcomes in assessing HDF safety, efficacy, and tolerance. For this purpose, we focus on cardiovascular stability and treatment tolerance, solute removal (phosphate, β2M), and inflammation, oxidative stress, and anemia.

5.1.1. Cardiovascular stability and treatment tolerance

In the short term, a significant reduction in the episodes of intradialytic hypotension was observed in HDF compared to conventional HD [16]. This has been ascribed to negative thermal balance (due to the infusion of relatively cool replacement fluid), a high sodium concentration of the substitution fluid, and/or removal of vasodilating mediators [4].

5.1.2. Solute removal: phosphate, β2-microglobulin

Several controlled studies have confirmed enhanced clearance and mass removal of β2M with HDF (30–40% higher than high-flux HD) accompanied by a 10 to 20% decline in circulating blood β2M concentrations [38, 39]. It must be reminded that reduction of circulating predialysis β2M takes time, as plasma levels reflect the equilibrium between production and elimination rates. Thus, 3 to 4 weeks are required to achieve a new steady-state and a serum concentration change [40]. Recently, it has been calculated in a large cohort of incident ESKD patients that each additional 10 L convection volume was associated with a 0.8 mg/L reduction of β2M [24].

Phosphate mass removal and serum phosphate is a major concern in ESKD patients. RRT accounts for 60 to 70% of the total amount of phosphate removed to restore weekly phosphate mass balance. The other 30 to 40% needs to be eliminated by feces through the combined action of diet and phosphate binders. Although still a matter of controversy, high efficiency HDF has been shown to enhance the phosphate mass removed by 15 to 20% [41] with a subsequent predialysis serum phosphate level reduction of 6%. The percentage of patients reaching target pretreatment serum phosphorus levels with HDF was reported to increase from 64 to 74% in the Convective Transport Study (CONTRAST) [42].

Higher clearances of a number of other uremic compounds have also been documented with HDF: complement factor D (a proinflammatory mediator), leptin (16 kDa; involved in loss of appetite), FGF23 (30 kDa, implicated in metabolic bone disorders and vascular calcification), various cytokines, circulating advanced glycosylation end products (AGEs), and AGE precursors [43, 44].

5.1.3. Inflammation, oxidative stress, and anemia

Inflammation and oxidative stress profiles tend to be improved in patients treated by HDF. Several prospective studies have shown that levels of C-reactive protein (CRP) and other sensitive biomarkers of inflammation (e.g., interleukin-6) and/or proinflammatory cells are reduced. In this field, the Rischio cardiovascolare nei pazienti afferenti all'area vasta in dialisi (RISCAVID) study is certainly one of the more convincing studies, being conducted in a large cohort of dialysis patients [7, 45]. A meta-analysis has recently reemphasized that the regular use of ultrapure dialysis fluid was the main driving force for such benefits [14].

The erythropoiesis-stimulating agent (ESA) dose could be reduced in HDF, as reported in several clinical studies and summarized in a systematic review [46]. The benefit was attributed to the combined effects of the higher removal of middle-sized toxins (erythropoietic inhibitor substances) and reduced inflammation due to the use of higher-quality water and dialysis fluid [47, 48]. However, this effect was not confirmed in a recent meta-analysis [49].

5.1.4. Clinical benefits

Several large cohort studies have indicated that the extended use of high-flux membranes and convective therapies has a beneficial impact on the development of β2M amyloidosis in the long term, reducing the incidence of carpal tunnel syndrome and other related manifestations [50, 51]. This beneficial effect probably results from the regular use of ultrapure water and biocompatible materials, reducing inflammation, combined with convective modalities that enhance β2M removal [52].

5.2. Endpoint outcomes (morbidity and mortality)

In this section, endpoint outcomes are hard primary outcomes in assessing HDF long-term efficacy. Consequently, the focus here is on mortality (all-cause and cardiovascular) and morbidity (hospitalization, dialysis-related pathology).

5.2.1. Observational (cohort) studies on hemodiafiltration and clinical endpoints

Locatelli et al. [50] conducted a retrospective observational study (Lombardy registry) of 6444 patients with ESKD who started RRT on HD, HDF, or hemofiltration (HF) between 1983 and 1995. A total of 1082 patients were treated with HDF or HF (first choice in the case of 188); the median follow-up time was 29.7 months. Interestingly, after adjustment for age, gender, and comorbidities (including diabetes), the RR for carpal tunnel surgery and mortality was 42% (statistically significant) and 10% lower (not statistically significant) in patients treated with HDF or HF.

In 2006, Canaud et al. [53] reported results of a prospective, nonrandomized observational study from the Dialysis Outcomes and Practice Patterns Study (DOPPS) of 2165 patients followed between 1998 and 2001 in five European countries. Patients were stratified into four groups: low-flux HD (n=1366), high-flux HD (n=546), low-efficiency HDF (n=156; substitution volume 5–14.9 L/treatment), and high-efficiency HDF (n=97; substitution volumes 15–24.9 L/treatment). Patient characteristics (including age and sex), 14 comorbidities, and time on dialysis were similar in each group. High-efficiency HDF patients had lower crude mortality rates than low-flux HD patients. After Cox regression analysis with adjustment, high-efficiency HDF patients had a 35% significantly lower mortality risk than those receiving low-flux HD.

Also in 2006, Jirka et al. published the results of an observational study of 2564 ESKD patients (394 on HDF) treated in Fresenius Medical Care clinics and followed for 12 months. Data were collected in the European Clinical Database (EuCliD) [54]. In this patient cohort, all-cause mortality was reduced by 43% and unadjusted mortality was reduced by 35% in patients treated with HDF compared to HD. Convection volume was not reported.

In 2008, Panichi et al. [7] reported the results of a prospective observational study performed in the northwestern part of Tuscany that included 757 ESKD patients (RISCAVID study) who were followed for 30 months. Treatment with low- or high-flux HD (n=424) was compared to treatment with HDF using substitution fluid delivered in bags (130 patients on low-volume HDF with acetate-free biofiltration (AFB) and 74 patients on HDF with convection volumes of

10–15 L/treatment) and treatment with online HDF (129 patients on HDF with convection volumes of 22–25 L/session). Cox proportional hazards regression analysis showed that online HDF and bag HDF patients had a significantly better survival than HD patients, having a 22% reduced risk of all-cause mortality after adjustment.

One year later, Vilar et al. [55] reported the results of an observational study of 858 incident ESKD patients in the United Kingdom followed over 18 years. Patients treated with online HDF (n=232) received 79% of treatments with this modality and a mean filtration volume of 14.9 L/session. The control group was treated exclusively with high-flux HD (n=626) and pure dialysis fluid. The mortality risk was significantly reduced in patients receiving predominantly HDF [hazard ratio (HR) 0.45; p<0.001] after adjustment for age, gender, body mass index, and comorbidities.

Imamovic et al. reported the Balkan experience in 2014. In this cohort study of 442 incident patients, the risk of death for HDF-treated patients relative to high-flux HD patients was 0.87 (nonsignificant) for low-volume HDF and 0.29 (highly significant) for high-volume HDF. After adjustment for covariates, the HR for patients on low-volume HDF remained statistically not significant compared to high-flux HD (HR 0.84; nonsignificant), whereas patients on high-volume HDF had a significantly lower HR (0.29; nonsignificant) than high-flux HD. In the time-dependent analysis, the mortality risk was not lower in high-volume HDF compared to high-flux HD (HR 0.48; nonsignificant), but this may be because 44% of the patients changed treatment modality during follow-up [56].

In 2015, Siriopol et al. published a report on the Romanian experience with HDF. In this study, the group of 221 prevalent patients treated with online HDF (mean convection volume was 22.2 L) was propensity score matched to a group of 431 patients treated with HD [57]. Online HDF was associated with a reduced mortality risk (HR 0.62; statistically significant). A second cohort consisting of 265 incident patients on HDF were matched with 530 patients treated with HD. The mortality risk was significantly lower in patients treated with HDF (HR 0.22; highly statistically significant).

In another study, Canaud et al. reported results based on the EuCliD database involving 1590 incident patients in 12 European countries. The patient groups receiving high volume HDF (≥21 L/session) were propensity score matched to the group receiving HD. Patients were followed for 2 years (HD group) or 1.6 years (high-volume HDF group) [58]. In this study, a nonsignificant survival advantage of HDF was found (HR 0.88; nonsignificant). Using inverse probability of censoring weighting (IPCW) to take bias due to the large amount of modality crossover during the follow-up time into consideration (7% HDF patients switched to HD; 55% HD patients switched to high-volume HDF), a statistically significant survival advantage of high-volume HDF was found (odds ratio 0.501; highly significant).

Canaud et al. [24] recently published the results of a dose-finding study exploring the optimal convection volume required to observe an increase in patient survival. This was a retrospective analysis involving 2293 incident HDF patients whose treatments were documented in the EuCliD database. Advanced statistical tools, including cubic spline analyses, were applied for the determination of the range of convection volume over which a survival benefit was observed. The relative survival rate of online HDF patients, adjusted for age, gender, comorbidities, vascular access, albumin, CRP, and dialysis dose, was found to increase at approximately 55L/week and to stay increased up to approximately 75L/week. Similar analysis of predialysis β2M concentrations found a nearly linear decrease in marker concentration, as convection volume increased from 40 to 75L/week. The analysis of log CRP levels showed a decrease over the same convection volume range.

Mercadal et al. reported a study using data from the French national Renal Epidemiology and Information Network (REIN) registry to assess the effects of HDF on mortality in the total population of incident dialysis patients (treatments were performed between 01/01/2008 and 31/12/2011 and patients were followed up to the end of 2012) [59]. Analyses were performed at both patient and facility levels. Here, 5526 out of 28,407 ESKD patients used HDF for a median of 1.2 years and 2254 of them used HDF exclusively. All-cause and cardiovascular mortality associated with HDF use were significantly reduced (HR 0.84 and 0.73, respectively). In patients treated exclusively with HDF, the beneficial effects on all-cause and cardiovascular mortality were more pronounced (HR 0.77 and 0.66, respectively). At the facility level, increasing the percentage of patients using HDF from 0 to 100% reduced the HR for all-cause and cardiovascular mortality (HR 0.87 and 0.72, respectively). The authors concluded that, irrespective of whether analyzed at patient or facility level, HDF treatment was associated with better survival.

5.2.2. Prospective RCTs

Four prospective controlled or randomized studies comparing HDF and standard HD have been reported in the past which were not designed (short term <12 months) or sufficiently powered (<100 patients) to assess mortality differences between modalities [25, 38, 60, 61]. These will not be discussed in this chapter.

The Dutch CONTRAST was performed in 29 centers in The Netherlands (n=26), Canada (n=2), and Norway (n=1) [62]. Here, 714 patients were randomized between treatment with low-flux HD and online postdilution HDF between 2004 and 2009, both with ultrapure dialysate. The primary endpoint was all-cause mortality, and the main secondary endpoint was a composite of fatal and nonfatal cardiovascular events. Of 358 HDF patients, 121 discontinued treatment during the study due to transplantation, switch to another center or therapy, or other reasons. Of 356 HD patients, 118 patients discontinued the allocated treatment. The mean follow-up was 36 months (range 5–79 months); during this period, 269 deaths occurred in 2170 person-years. All-cause mortality (HR 0.95; nonsignificant) as well as cardiovascular events (fatal and nonfatal; HR 1.07; nonsignificant) were not affected by treatment modality. Although the target convection volume was set at 24 L/treatment, the mean volume achieved was 20.7 L/session and only one third of centers achieved at least 24 L/session. Post hoc analyses based on convection volume delivered (tertiles) showed a significantly lower mortality in patients receiving the highest convection volume (>21.95 L/session). In this subgroup, mortality risk was reduced by 39% compared to HD (HR 0.61; significant), which remained after extensive adjustments.

The Turkish Hemodiafiltration Study with 782 patients was conducted between 2007 and 2010 in 10 centers; patients were randomized to treatment with online postdilution HDF or high-flux HD [63]. Patients with central venous catheters, poor blood flow, and significant residual urine output were excluded. The primary endpoint was a composite of all-cause mortality and first nonfatal cardiovascular event. Of 391 patients treated with HDF, 110 discontinued the study (28%), including 40 (10%) who terminated early due to vascular access problems. Of 391 patients randomized to HD, 90 patients (23%) dropped out. The mean follow-up time was 23 months (range 1–38 months). The mean substitution volume was 17.2 L/session and the mean intradialytic weight gain was 2.4 L/treatment, corresponding to a mean total convection volume of 19.6 L/treatment. The RR of death and first cardiovascular event was 0.82 (nonsignificant), and the RR for all-cause and cardiovascular mortality was 0.79 (nonsignificant) and 0.72 (nonsignificant), respectively. In a post hoc analysis, patients who achieved a convection volume above the median of 17.4 L/session had a significant lower risk of all-cause and cardiovascular mortality (RR 0.54 and 0.29, respectively; both highly significant). This association remained after extensive adjustments for age, gender, comorbidity, and practice patterns.

The Catalonian Hemodiafiltration Study (ESHOL) included 906 Spanish dialysis patients in 27 units who were randomized to online postdilution HDF (n=456) and HD (n=450) [64]. In the HD group, 8% of the patients were treated with low-flux membranes and 92% were treated with high-flux membranes. The mean follow-up time was 23 months. Here, 355 patients dropped out of the study for various reasons and were censored at the time of loss (36% in the HD group and 42% in the HDF group). Centers involved in the study received a short training course on how to achieve the targeted convection volume. The median convection volume in HDF treated patients was 22.9 to 23.9 L/treatment. Here, 207 events were observed in 1730 patient-years. A significant 30% decrease in all-cause mortality and 33% decrease in cardiovascular mortality were observed in the HDF group. Interestingly, a post hoc analysis based on convection volume showed that the highest convection volume tertile (>25.4 L/treatment) was associated with a lower mortality risk (HR 0.55; highly significant) compared to HD patients.

5.2.3. *Meta-analyses*

Several meta-analyses comparing conventional HD and convective-based therapies have been published over the last decade.

Rabindranath et al. from the Cochrane group performed two analyses in 2005 and 2006. The latter included 20 trials (657 patients). Mortality results were available only in 4 trials (336 patients) and different therapies were mixed (AFB, HF, and HDF). The authors found no difference in mortality risk for patients treated with convective-based therapies [26, 65]. This systematic review was severely criticized due to its poor methodology [66, 67].

Susantitaphong et al. [49] compared convective-based therapies to standard low-flux HD. HF, HDF, AFB, and high-flux HD were all included in the convective therapy group. This meta-analysis aggregated data of 12,182 patients. Convective therapies resulted in a nonsignificant decrease in all-cause mortality (RR 0.88) and all-cause hospitalization (RR 0.91); a significant decrease in therapy-related hypotension (RR 0.55) and cardiovascular mortality (RR 0.84) was reported. The authors concluded that convective therapies were associated with improved clearance of uremic solutes, but the potential long-term benefits of specific convective modalities could not be confirmed.

Wang et al. [68] conducted a systematic review and meta-analysis that included 16 trials and 3220 patients treated with convective-based therapies (HDF and HF) and with standard HD (low- and high-flux). Convection volume was not considered as a confounder in this analysis. On the one hand, the authors concluded that convective modalities did not significantly reduce the risk of cardiovascular events (RR 0.85) or all-cause mortality (RR 0.83). On the other hand, they noted that convective modalities reduced intradialytic symptomatic hypotension (RR 0.49) and reduced serum β2M levels (-5.95 mg/L).

Mostovaya et al. [69] compared exclusively HDF to HD (low- and high-flux) including 2402 patients. The meta-analysis identified six RCTs. The convective arm consisted exclusively of HDF patients treated with different HDF modes (a mixture of postdilution, mid-dilution, and predilution HDF, and of online HDF and HDF with bags) and achieving a specified minimum convection volume. All-cause and cardiovascular mortality were reduced with HDF compared to HD (RR 0.8 and 0.73, respectively).

Nistor et al. [70, 71] from the Cochrane group updated the previous systematic review of 2005 and compared HD (low- and high-flux) to convective-based modalities (HF, AFB, bag HDF, and online HDF) without considering convection volume. Thirty-five trials (4039 patients) were included in this meta-analysis and the effects on mortality were estimated. The convective group consisted of 1648 patients, but 227 of them were treated with low convection volumes. Within the limitations of the review (e.g., studies reviewed were partially old and referred to a diverse mixture of HDF modalities), the authors concluded that convective therapies had no significant effect on reducing all-cause mortality (RR 0.87), cardiovascular mortality (RR 0.75), and intradialytic hypotension (RR 0.72) but had uncertain effects on nonfatal cardiovascular events (RR 1.14) and hospitalization (RR 1.21).

5.2.4. Individual participant data meta-analysis

An alternative to the aggregated data meta-analysis approach is to perform meta-analysis of individual participant data in which the raw "individual level data" for each study are obtained and analyzed. The term "individual participant data" relates to the data recorded for each participant in a study. Individual participant data sets of four randomized trials were pooled and used to compare online HDF to HD. The four studies aggregated 2793 patients and were designed to examine the effects of HDF on mortality endpoints. Bias by informative censoring of patients was resolved. HRs comparing the effect of online HDF versus HD on all-cause and cause-specific mortality were calculated using Cox proportional hazard regression models.

In the first part of this individual participant data meta-analysis, Davenport et al. [72] analyzed the relationship between convection volume and patient outcomes. After a median follow-up time of 2.5 years, 769 of the 2793 participants had died (292 cardiovascular deaths). Convection volumes were either not standardized or standardized to weight, body mass index, body surface area, and total body water. Data were analyzed by multivariable Cox proportional hazards modeling from 2793 patients. All-cause mortality was reduced when the convective dose was unstandardized or standardized to body surface area or total body water; corresponding HRs were 0.65 (0.51–0.82), 0.74 (0.58–0.93), and 0.71 (0.56–0.93). Standardization by body weight or body mass index was not associated with significant survival advantages. Higher convection volumes were generally associated with greater survival benefit with online HDF, but results varied across the different ways of standardization for body size. Further studies should take body size into account when evaluating the impact of convection volume on mortality endpoints.

In the second part of this analysis, Peters et al. [73] also investigated the effects of convection volume on patient outcomes. HRs comparing the effect of online HDF versus HD on all-cause and cause-specific mortality were calculated using Cox proportional hazards regression models. The relationship between convection volume and the study outcomes was examined by delivered convection volume standardized to body surface area. Online HDF reduced the risk of all-cause mortality by 14% and cardiovascular mortality by 23%. There was no evidence for a differential effect in predefined convection volume subgroups. The largest survival benefit was for patients receiving the highest delivered convection volume (>23 L/1.73 m^2 body surface area per session), with a multivariable-adjusted HR of 0.78 (95% confidence interval 0.62–0.98) for all-cause mortality and 0.69 for cardiovascular disease mortality. This pooled individual participant analysis indicates that online HDF reduces the risk of mortality in ESKD patients. This effect holds across a variety of important convection volume subgroups of patients and is most pronounced for those receiving a higher convection volume normalized to body surface area.

6. Conclusions

Online HDF can no longer be considered an experimental treatment; it is a mature RRT that is applied daily to sustain the lives of more than 160,000 ESKD patients worldwide, including 80,000 in Europe, Middle East, and Africa. Europe has played a leading role in developing this therapy, where the prevalence of HDF is close to 18% with variations across countries from 0 to 100%.

Interestingly, it has recently been also shown that clinical benefits associated with HDF were directly correlated with the total ultrafiltered volume delivered, either per session or per week. This finding adds a new component, namely convective dose, that needs to be integrated into our conventional dialysis adequacy concept. In addition, accumulating evidence from both retrospective and prospective RCT studies confirm the clinical safety and sustainability of HDF therapy and support its superiority over conventional HD in terms of morbidity and mortality.

In line with these facts, the remaining and crucial challenges today are to implement best clinical practices to achieve the optimal convective dose required, to define which subset of ESKD patients should benefit most, and to evaluate new tools facilitating and fine-tuning HDF prescription according to ESKD patient needs (e.g., electrolyte balancing and quantification and homeostasis).

7. Compliance with ethical standards

Conflict of interest: Bernard Canaud, Aileen Grassmann, Laura Scatizzi, and Daniele Marcelli are employees of Fresenius Medical Care.

Author details

Bernard Canaud[1*], Aileen Grassmann[2], Laura Scatizzi[2] and Daniele Marcelli[2]

*Address all correspondence to: bernard.canaud@fmc-ag.com

1 Center of Excellence Medical, Fresenius Medical Care, Bad Homburg, Germany

2 Clinical and Epidemiological Research, Fresenius Medical Care, Bad Homburg, Germany

References

[1] Canaud B, Chenine L, Henriet D, Leray H. Cross-membrane flux is a major factor influencing dialysis patient outcomes. Contrib Nephrol. 2008;161:178–84.

[2] Maduell F, Navarro V, Cruz MC, Torregrosa E, Garcia D, Simon V, et al. Osteocalcin and myoglobin removal in on-line hemodiafiltration versus low- and high-flux hemodialysis. Am J Kidney Dis. 2002;40(3):582–9.

[3] Kanamori T, Mizoguchi K. Solute-removal enhancement caused by local convective flow in a hemodialyzer. J Artif Organs. 2012;15(3):305–10.

[4] van der Sande FM, Kooman JP, Konings CJ, Leunissen KM. Thermal effects and blood pressure response during postdilution hemodiafiltration and hemodialysis: the effect of amount of replacement fluid and dialysate temperature. J Am Soc Nephrol. 2001;12(9):1916–20.

[5] Daugirdas JT. Lower cardiovascular mortality with high–volume hemodiafiltration: a cool effect? Nephrol Dial Transplant. 2015. doi: 10.1093/ndt/gfv412.

[6] Ramirez R, Martin-Malo A, Aljama P. Inflammation and hemodiafiltration. Contrib Nephrol. 2007;158:210–5.

[7] Panichi V, Rizza GM, Paoletti S, Bigazzi R, Aloisi M, Barsotti G, et al. Chronic inflammation and mortality in haemodialysis: effect of different renal replacement therapies. Results from the RISCAVID study. Nephrol Dial Transplant. 2008;23(7):2337–43.

[8] den Hoedt CH, Bots ML, Grooteman MP, van der Weerd NC, Mazairac AH, Penne EL, et al. Online hemodiafiltration reduces systemic inflammation compared to low-flux hemodialysis. Kidney Int. 2014;86(2):423–32.

[9] Canaud B, Bowry SK. Emerging clinical evidence on online hemodiafiltration: does volume of ultrafiltration matter? Blood Purif. 2013;35(1–3):55–62.

[10] Bowry SK, Canaud B. Achieving high convective volumes in on-line hemodiafiltration. Blood Purif. 2013;35 Suppl 1:23–8.

[11] Chapdelaine I, de Roij van Zuijdewijn CL, Mostovaya IM, Levesque R, Davenport A, Blankestijn PJ, et al. Optimization of the convection volume in online post-dilution haemodiafiltration: practical and technical issues. Clin Kidney J. 2015;8(2):191–8.

[12] Chapdelaine I, Mostovaya IM, Blankestijn PJ, Bots ML, van den Dorpel MA, Levesque R, et al. Treatment policy rather than patient characteristics determines convection volume in online post-dilution hemodiafiltration. Blood Purif. 2014;37(3):229–37.

[13] Honda H, Suzuki H, Hosaka N, Hirai Y, Sanada D, Nakamura M, et al. Ultrapure dialysate influences serum myeloperoxidase levels and lipid metabolism. Blood Purif. 2009;28(1):29–39.

[14] Susantitaphong P, Riella C, Jaber BL. Effect of ultrapure dialysate on markers of inflammation, oxidative stress, nutrition and anemia parameters: a meta-analysis. Nephrol Dial Transplant. 2013;28(2):438–46.

[15] Movilli E, Camerini C, Gaggia P, Zubani R, Feller P, Salviani C, et al. Total convection affects serum beta2 microglobulin and C-reactive protein but not erythropoietin requirement following post-dilutional hemodiafiltration. Am J Nephrol. 2015;41(6): 494–501.

[16] Locatelli F, Altieri P, Andrulli S, Bolasco P, Sau G, Pedrini LA, et al. Hemofiltration and hemodiafiltration reduce intradialytic hypotension in ESRD. J Am Soc Nephrol. 2010;21(10):1798–807.

[17] Kooman J, Basci A, Pizzarelli F, Canaud B, Haage P, Fouque D, et al. EBPG guideline on haemodynamic instability. Nephrol Dial Transplant. 2007;22 Suppl 2:ii22–44.

[18] Kooman JP, Sande FM, Leunissen KML. Hemodynamic stability and cardiovascular effects of convective therapies. In: Nubé JM, Grooteman PCM, Blankestijn P, editors. Hemodiafiltration: Theory, Technology and Clinical Practice. Cham: Springer International Publishing; 2016. p. 215–31.

[19] Maduell F, Arias M, Duran CE, Vera M, Fontsere N, Azqueta M, et al. Nocturnal, every-other-day, online haemodiafiltration: an effective therapeutic alternative. Nephrol Dial Transplant. 2012;27(4):1619–31.

[20] Cornelis T, van der Sande FM, Eloot S, Cardinaels E, Bekers O, Damoiseaux J, et al. Acute hemodynamic response and uremic toxin removal in conventional and extended hemodialysis and hemodiafiltration: a randomized crossover study. Am J Kidney Dis. 2014;64(2):247–56.

[21] Canaud B, Bowry SK. Revisiting frontiers of tolerability and efficacy in renal replacement therapy. Am J Kidney Dis. 2014;64(2):171–3.

[22] Tattersall JE, Ward RA. Online haemodiafiltration: definition, dose quantification and safety revisited. Nephrol Dial Transplant. 2013;28(3):542–50.

[23] Grooteman MPC, Nubé MJ, Bots ML. Clinical trials on hemodiafiltration. In: Nubé MJ, Grooteman MPC, Blankestijn P, editors. Hemodiafiltration: Theory, Technology and Clinical Practice. Switzerland: Springer International Publishing; 2015. pp. 199–213.

[24] Canaud B, Barbieri C, Marcelli D, Bellocchio F, Bowry S, Mari F, et al. Optimal convection volume for improving patient outcomes in an international incident dialysis cohort treated with online hemodiafiltration. Kidney Int. 2015;88(5):1108–16.

[25] Kerr PB, Argiles A, Flavier JL, Canaud B, Mion CM. Comparison of hemodialysis and hemodiafiltration: a long-term longitudinal study. Kidney Int. 1992;41(4):1035–40.

[26] Rabindranath KS, Strippoli GF, Roderick P, Wallace SA, MacLeod AM, Daly C. Comparison of hemodialysis, hemofiltration, and acetate-free biofiltration for ESRD: systematic review. Am J Kidney Dis. 2005;45(3):437–47.

[27] Tsobanelis T, Hensel N, Sierp O, Kollia M, Kurz P. Improving patient care through reduced complexity in haemodiafiltration: a comparative analysis of two haemodialysis machines. Abstract submitted to the 53rd Congress ERA-EDTA, Vienna, Austria, May 21–24. 2016;16-A-1698.

[28] Tsobanelis T, Hensel N, Kollia M, Sierp O, Kurz P. Haemodiafiltration relative infection risk: a comparative analysis of two dialysis machines. Abstract submitted to the 53rd Congress ERA-EDTA, Vienna, Austria, May 21–24. 2016;16-A-1795.

[29] Schleser A, Fleck N, Tsobanelis T. The impact of disposables towards more eco-friendly and less costly haemodialysis. Abstract submitted to the 53rd Congress ERA-EDTA, Vienna, Austria, May 21–24. 2016;16-A-337.

[30] Canaud B, Ledebo I. History and current status of online haemodiafiltration. In: Nubé JM, Grooteman PCM, Blankestijn P, editors. Hemodiafiltration: Theory, Technology and Clinical Practice. Cham: Springer International Publishing; 2016. pp. 1–16.

[31] Ronco C, Clarke WR. Hollow-fiber dialyzers: technical and clinical considerations. In: Nissenson AR, Fine RN, editors. Clinical Dialysis, Fourth Edition. New York: McGraw-Hill Education; 2005.

[32] Pedrini LA, Ponti R, Faranna P, Cozzi G, Locatelli F. Sodium modeling in hemodiafiltration. Kidney Int. 1991 Sep;40(3):525–32.

[33] Pedrini LA, De Cristofaro V, Pagliari B, Ruggiero P. Dialysate/infusate composition and infusion mode in on-line hemodiafiltration. In: Ronco C, Greca GL, editors. Hemodialysis Technology. Contributions to Nephrology. Basel: Karger; 2002. pp. 344–9.

[34] Malberti F, Ravani P. The choice of the dialysate calcium concentration in the management of patients on haemodialysis and haemodiafiltration. Nephrol Dial Transplant. 2003;18 Suppl 7:vii37–40; discussion vii57.

[35] Bacchetta J, Sellier-Leclerc AL, Bertholet-Thomas A, Carlier MC, Cartier R, Cochat P, et al. Calcium balance in pediatric online hemodiafiltration: beware of sodium and bicarbonate in the dialysate. Nephrol Ther. 2015;11(6):483–6.

[36] Havlin J, Schuck O, Charvat J, Slaby K, Horackova M, Klaboch J, et al. Acid-base disorders associated with serum electrolyte patterns in patients on hemodiafiltration. Nephrol Ther. 2015;11(7):551–7.

[37] Pedrini LA, De CV, Pagliari B. Effects of the infusion mode on bicarbonate balance in on-line hemodiafiltration. Int J Artif Organs. 2002;25(2):100–6.

[38] Ward RA, Schmidt B, Hullin J, Hillebrand GF, Samtleben W. A comparison of on-line hemodiafiltration and high-flux hemodialysis: a prospective clinical study. J Am Soc Nephrol. 2000;11(12):2344–50.

[39] Pedrini LA, Gmerek A, Wagner J. Efficiency of post-dilution hemodiafiltration with a high-flux alpha-polysulfone dialyzer. Int J Artif Organs. 2011;34(5):397–404.

[40] Canaud B, Assounga A, Flavier JL, Slingeneyer A, Aznar R, Robinet-Levy M, et al. Beta-2 microglobulin serum levels in maintenance dialysis. What does it mean? ASAIO Trans. 1988;34(4):923–9.

[41] Lornoy W, De Meester J, Becaus I, Billiouw JM, Van Malderen PA, Van Pottelberge M. Impact of convective flow on phosphorus removal in maintenance hemodialysis patients. J Ren Nutr. 2006;16(1):47–53.

[42] Penne EL, van der Weerd NC, van den Dorpel MA, Grooteman MP, Levesque R, Nube MJ, et al. Short-term effects of online hemodiafiltration on phosphate control: a result from the randomized controlled Convective Transport Study (CONTRAST). Am J Kidney Dis. 2010;55(1):77–87.

[43] Lin CL, Huang CC, Yu CC, Yang HY, Chuang FR, Yang CW. Reduction of advanced glycation end product levels by on-line hemodiafiltration in long-term hemodialysis patients. Am J Kidney Dis. 2003;42(3):524–31.

[44] Stein G, Franke S, Mahiout A, Schneider S, Sperschneider H, Borst S, et al. Influence of dialysis modalities on serum AGE levels in end-stage renal disease patients. Nephrol Dial Transplant. 2001;16(5):999–1008.

[45] Desideri G, Panichi V, Paoletti S, Grassi D, Bigazzi R, Beati S, et al. Soluble CD40 ligand is predictive of combined cardiovascular morbidity and mortality in patients on haemodialysis at a relatively short-term follow-up. Nephrol Dial Transplant. 2011;26(9):2983–8.

[46] Bowry SK, Gatti E. Impact of hemodialysis therapy on anemia of chronic kidney disease: the potential mechanisms. Blood Purif. 2011;32(3):210–9.

[47] Panichi V, Rosati A, Bigazzi R, Paoletti S, Mantuano E, Beati S, et al. Anaemia and resistance to erythropoiesis-stimulating agents as prognostic factors in haemodialysis patients: results from the RISCAVID study. Nephrol Dial Transplant. 2011;26(8):2641–8.

[48] Panichi V, Scatena A, Rosati A, Giusti R, Ferro G, Malagnino E, et al. High-volume online haemodiafiltration improves erythropoiesis-stimulating agent (ESA) resistance in comparison with low-flux bicarbonate dialysis: results of the REDERT study. Nephrol Dial Transplant. 2015;30(4):682–9.

[49] Susantitaphong P, Siribamrungwong M, Jaber BL. Convective therapies versus low-flux hemodialysis for chronic kidney failure: a meta-analysis of randomized controlled trials. Nephrol Dial Transplant. 2013;28(11):2859–74.

[50] Locatelli F, Marcelli D, Conte F, Limido A, Malberti F, Spotti D. Comparison of mortality in ESRD patients on convective and diffusive extracorporeal treatments. The Registro Lombardo Dialisi E Trapianto. Kidney Int. 1999;55(1):286–93.

[51] Nakai S, Iseki K, Tabei K, Kubo K, Masakane I, Fushimi K, et al. Outcomes of hemodiafiltration based on Japanese dialysis patient registry. Am J Kidney Dis. 2001;384 Suppl 1:S212–6.

[52] Schiffl H. Impact of advanced dialysis technology on the prevalence of dialysis-related amyloidosis in long-term maintenance dialysis patients. Hemodial Int. 2014;18(1):136–41.

[53] Canaud B, Bragg-Gresham JL, Marshall MR, Desmeules S, Gillespie BW, Depner T, et al. Mortality risk for patients receiving hemodiafiltration versus hemodialysis: European results from the DOPPS. Kidney Int. 2006;69(11):2087–93.

[54] Jirka T, Cesare S, Di Benedetto A, Perera Chang M, Ponce P, Richards N, et al. Mortality risk for patients receiving hemodiafiltration versus hemodialysis. Kidney Int. 2006;70(8):1524; author reply 1525.

[55] Vilar E, Fry AC, Wellsted D, Tattersall JE, Greenwood RN, Farrington K. Long-term outcomes in online hemodiafiltration and high-flux hemodialysis: a comparative analysis. Clin J Am Soc Nephrol. 2009;4(12):1944–53.

[56] Imamovic G, Hrvacevic R, Kapun S, Marcelli D, Bayh I, Grassmann A, et al. Survival of incident patients on high-volume online hemodiafiltration compared to low-volume online hemodiafiltration and high-flux hemodialysis. Int Urol Nephrol. 2014;46(6): 1191–200.

[57] Siriopol D, Canaud B, Stuard S, Mircescu G, Nistor I, Covic A. New insights into the effect of haemodiafiltration on mortality: the Romanian experience. Nephrol Dial Transplant. 2015;30(2):294–301.

[58] Canaud B, Bayh I, Marcelli D, Ponce P, Merello JI, Gurevich K, et al. Improved survival of incident patients with high-volume haemodiafiltration: a propensity-matched cohort study with inverse probability of censoring weighting. Nephron. 2015;129(3): 179–88.

[59] Mercadal L, Franck JE, Metzger M, Urena Torres P, de Cornelissen F, Edet S, et al. Hemodiafiltration versus hemodialysis and survival in patients with ESRD: the French Renal Epidemiology and Information Network (REIN) Registry. Am J Kidney Dis. 2015. pii: S0272-6386(15)01436-5. doi: 10.1053/j.ajkd.2015.11.016.

[60] Wizemann V, Lotz C, Techert F, Uthoff S. On-line haemodiafiltration versus low-flux haemodialysis. A prospective randomized study. Nephrol Dial Transplant. 2000;15 Suppl 1:43–8.

[61] Schiffl H. Prospective randomized cross-over long-term comparison of online haemodiafiltration and ultrapure high-flux haemodialysis. Eur J Med Res. 2007;12(1):26–33.

[62] Grooteman MP, van den Dorpel MA, Bots ML, Penne EL, van der Weerd NC, Mazairac AH, et al. Effect of online hemodiafiltration on all-cause mortality and cardiovascular outcomes. J Am Soc Nephrol. 2012;23(6):1087–96.

[63] Ok E, Asci G, Toz H, Ok ES, Kircelli F, Yilmaz M, et al. Mortality and cardiovascular events in online haemodiafiltration (OL-HDF) compared with high-flux dialysis: results from the Turkish OL-HDF Study. Nephrol Dial Transplant. 2013;28(1):192–202.

[64] Maduell F, Moreso F, Pons M, Ramos R, Mora-Macia J, Carreras J, et al. High-efficiency postdilution online hemodiafiltration reduces all-cause mortality in hemodialysis patients. J Am Soc Nephrol. 2013;24(3):487–97.

[65] Rabindranath KS, Strippoli GF, Daly C, Roderick PJ, Wallace S, MacLeod AM. Haemodiafiltration, haemofiltration and haemodialysis for end-stage kidney disease. Cochrane Database Syst Rev. 2006(4):CD006258.

[66] Locatelli F. Comparison of hemodialysis, hemodiafiltration, and hemofiltration: systematic review or systematic error? Am J Kidney Dis. 2005;46(4):787–8; author reply 788–9.

[67] Wizemann V. Si tacuisses. Am J Kidney Dis. 2005;46(4):787; author reply 788–9.

[68] Wang AY, Ninomiya T, Al-Kahwa A, Perkovic V, Gallagher MP, Hawley C, et al. Effect of hemodiafiltration or hemofiltration compared with hemodialysis on mortality and cardiovascular disease in chronic kidney failure: a systematic review and meta-analysis of randomized trials. Am J Kidney Dis. 2014;63(6):968–78.

[69] Mostovaya IM, Blankestijn PJ, Bots ML, Covic A, Davenport A, Grooteman MP, et al. Clinical evidence on hemodiafiltration: a systematic review and a meta-analysis. Semin Dial. 2014;27(2):119–27.

[70] Nistor I, Palmer SC, Craig JC, Saglimbene V, Vecchio M, Covic A, et al. Convective versus diffusive dialysis therapies for chronic kidney failure: an updated systematic review of randomized controlled trials. Am J Kidney Dis. 2014;63(6):954–67.

[71] Nistor I, Palmer SC, Craig JC, Saglimbene V, Vecchio M, Covic A, et al. Haemodiafiltration, haemofiltration and haemodialysis for end-stage kidney disease. Cochrane Database Syst Rev. 2015;5:CD006258.

[72] Davenport A, Peters SA, Bots ML, Canaud B, Grooteman MP, Asci G, et al. Higher convection volume exchange with online hemodiafiltration is associated with survival advantage for dialysis patients: the effect of adjustment for body size. Kidney Int. 2016;89(1):193–199. doi:10.1038/ki.2015.264.

[73] Peters SA, Bots ML, Canaud B, Davenport A, Grooteman MP, Kircelli F, et al. Haemodiafiltration and mortality in end–stage kidney disease patients: a pooled individual participant data analysis from four randomized controlled trials. Nephrol Dial Transplant. 2015. doi: 10.1093/ndt/gfv349.

Chapter 7

Home Haemodialysis and Haemodiafiltration

Sandip Mitra and Kunaal Kharbanda

Additional information is available at the end of the chapter

http://dx.doi.org/10.5772/64095

Abstract

There has been a resurgence in home haemodialysis over the last decade and interest in online haemodiafiltration in gaining momentum with advances in technology and the results of recent clinical trials. Both increasing haemodialysis frequency and treatment time have a number of potential benefits in improving dialysis efficiency and are ideally placed in the home setting. This chapter describes the rationale behind dialysis treatments, which go beyond conventional haemodialysis (CHD) and future avenues for home dialysis, which may involve combining convective therapy with more frequent treatment.

Keywords: haemodialysis, haemodiafiltration, extended haemodialysis, home haemodialysis

1. Introduction

Haemodialysis treatment has changed the lives of millions of patients around the world who have advanced kidney disease. The treatment has advanced considerably since the first treatment on a human, lasting just 15 minutes and performed by George Haas in Giessen, Germany, in October 1924 [1]. It was not until the 1960s when maintenance haemodialysis really started and at present, over 90 years since Haas, there are over 400,000 prevalent users in the USA alone [2]. Dialysis provides a bridge to transplantation for some, and for others, it allows survival when residual kidney function is no longer sufficient to sustain life. While the survival of patients has improved since the early days of its inception, the survival of haemodialysis patients remains unacceptably poor. In the United Kingdom, 18% of those aged 65–74 starting haemodialysis will not survive 1 year [3]. Five-year survival data has often been compared to those of patients with cancer to make the figures more tangible. With recent figures showing 50% survival at 5.8 years in the 55–64 years group [4], it is not hard to see why this comparison is made. Clearly, one of the key challenges for the nephrology community is to change this unacceptably high mortality rate. In addition to this, there are many other factors that make a large difference to the patient in front of us, and arguably, these are as important to address and considerably improve.

2. Background

The aim of haemodialysis is to replicate normal physiology as much as possible. Although this may sound straightforward initially, there are a vast array of factors to consider. The ideal treatment should give good survival rates, prevent cardiovascular events and hospitalizations, effectively manage fluid and salt balance and address the anaemia and mineral-bone disorder associated with chronic kidney disease (CKD). Patient well-being, cognition, sleep, the ability to work and nutritional status are also hugely important factors which need addressing and the list could continue. For a treatment, which for the majority of patients is performed for 12 hours of the week (just 7% of the week in terms of time), this is an incredibly tall order and it is not entirely surprising that outcomes remain poor.

Conventional haemodialysis (CHD) is the most common treatment schedule and lasts for 3–4 hours thrice weekly. This treatment mainly takes place in a hospital or in a dedicated dialysis unit. Other treatment regimes include short daily haemodialysis (SDHD), which is performed for 1.5–3 hours 5–7 times per week, long nocturnal daily haemodialysis (LNDHD) which is performed for 6–8 hours 5–7 times per week and long conventional haemodialysis (LHD), which is typically 8 hours 3 times per week.

Although CHD is the most common treatment regime now, LHD was the most common treatment initially in the 1960s [5]. This treatment came about purely by convention. Home haemodialysis in the United Kingdom was started in London in 1964 by Shaldon and his team [6] and expanded following this. Home haemodialysis was necessary as hospital facilities were sparse, treatment times were lengthy and home dialysis offered both financial and logistical benefit. Prevalence in the United Kingdom peaked in 1982 when 62% of HD patients were at home [3]. As dialysis treatment time shortened and patient numbers increased, haemodialysis practice changed from a predominantly home-based therapy to a predominantly hospital-based therapy.

The National Cooperative Dialysis Study (NCDS) ($n = 151$) [7] was published in 1981. It showed no difference between the shorter and longer duration dialysis groups (2.5–3.5 hours three times per week vs. 4.5–5 hours three times per week). This further paved the way to the adoption of CHD. Data from this study were later used to develop a method for calculating haemodialysis adequacy [8] K_t/V_{urea} (K_t/V) which is now used worldwide. K_t/V exclusively looks at small molecule clearance as a marker of dialysis adequacy. There is an association between dialysis dose and mortality [9]; however, the benefit (from the NCDS data) was seen up until a K_t/V of 1.2 with no survival advantage with doses above this. This was later echoed in the much larger HEMO study (involving 1846 patients) and again showed no advantage in increasing the dialysis dose above a K_t/V of 1.3. Dialysis treatment time was not investigated in this study.

It would seem therefore that with K_t/V we have reached a ceiling where improvements can no longer be made within the restrictions of a thrice weekly schedule, and we must start looking at other ways to improve outcomes in haemodialysis. The most significant causes of death in haemodialysis patients are cardiovascular in nature and this has been well known for some time. UK registry data show that almost a third of deaths in dialysis patients are cardiovascular in nature [4]. It is also clear that the two-day gap in CHD is harmful with all-cause and cardiovascular mortality being higher on the day after the long interval [10]. Further data show the highest rate of cardiovascular events in the first month after starting haemodialysis and a high-risk period extending to 4 months [11].

Based on all of this, a strong argument can be made to further explore more frequent and extended haemodialysis treatments.

3. Extracorporeal dialysis therapy

The basic principle behind dialysis is the removal of solutes across a semipermeable membrane. Haemodialysis relies on the process of diffusion where solutes move from an area of high concentration to an area of low concentration. Solutes pass from the patients' blood to the dialysis fluid across the dialysis membrane in this manner. The concentration gradient is maintained by the countercurrent flow of dialysate and blood and the maintenance of adequate blood and dialysate flow.

Haemofiltration allows the clearance of larger molecules through the process of convection. A hydrostatic pressure gradient is used to pass the patient's blood across a membrane with a large pore size. Solutes follow water through a process called "solvent drag" [12]. Large volumes of fluid are typically filtered and a replacement fluid is required, which enters the dialysis circuit and is mixed with the patient's blood before it is returned.

Haemodiafiltration (HDF) combines the techniques of both haemodialysis and haemofiltration. Solutes are cleared by both diffusion and convection, thus allowing more efficient clearance of both small and middle molecules. The replacement fluid can either be obtained from pre-prepared bags or prepared "online" by the machine (OL-HDF), which is able to produce ultrapure fluid. This dialysis therapy has a number of potential advantages, which are discussed in more detail later in this chapter.

3.1. Clearance in extracorporeal dialysis

K_t/V is widely used to give us information on dialysis adequacy; however, it is solely dependent on the clearance of urea. Urea has the advantage of being easy to measure; however, it may not be directly toxic and many of the identified uraemic toxins are larger in size and are not cleared efficiently by conventional haemodialysis [13]. In general, molecules are classified as small molecular weight (MW) molecules (<500 Da), middle MW molecules (>500 Da) and protein-bound molecules. β2-microglobulin (B2M), which is commonly used as a marker of middle molecules, has a molecular weight of around 11,800 Da. It has been demonstrated that outcomes are improved when middle molecular clearance (1000–50,000 Da in the study) are enhanced [14]. There has been much interest in increasing middle MW molecule clearance, and it is clear that accumulation of middle MW molecules can be harmful such as in the case of B2M which can lead to dialysis-related amyloidosis [15].

β-Trace protein, cystatin-C and B2M are all middle MW molecules that are freely filtered, resorbed and catabolized in the tubular cells. A study by Lindström et al. [16] has shown clear differences in the clearance of these molecules by different dialysis modalities—CHD did not change the concentrations of any of these proteins while in HDF both cystatin C and B2M were reduced and β-trace protein was only reduced in HDF. This demonstrates a clear difference between dialysis modalities in terms of clearance and a clear biomarker that could be measured. Moreover, β-trace protein had been found to be an independent predictor of both death and cardiovascular mortality in haemodialysis patients [17]. The use of such molecules could be part of the way that we assess haemodialysis adequacy in the future and tailor treatment to the patient.

3.2. Biocompatibilty in dialysis

The specifications of dialysis membranes have improved considerably. The use of cellulose-based membranes were common initially; however, they were associated with complement and leucocyte activation [18] resulting in dialyser reactions. The majority of dialysis membranes in use now are synthetic and are more biocompatible—reactions can still occur however and anaphylactoid reactions have been reported, particularly in patients on ACE inhibitors [19]. More recently, dialysis membranes have been manufactured with larger pore sizes to allow a higher ultrafiltration rate and allow clearance of larger molecules. Membranes can be classified as high flux or low flux and for the purposes of the HEMO study [20] were defined as B2M clearances of <10 ml/min for low flux and >20 ml/min for high flux. High-flux membranes have been found to lower pre-dialysis B2M concentrations [21] and may prevent dialysis-related amyloidosis [22]. Several observational studies have identified a survival benefit with high-flux dialysers [23, 24]. Although the HEMO study showed no benefit from high-flux membranes, the study may not have been sufficiently powered to detect a significant benefit [25]. The subsequent European study, the MPO Study [26], showed survival benefit to those patients with a serum albumin of <40 g/l. Several guidelines now recommend high-flux dialysers including the European Renal Association [27] and practice has also changed considerably.

The production of a high-quality infusion fluid is of paramount importance in HDF. More than 20 litres of infusion fluid can be administered to the patient during a typical HDF session and thus ultrapure water and dialysis fluid are required. Ultrapure water is defined by the standard for replacement fluid requiring <0.1 colony-forming units (CFU)/ml and an endotoxin concentration <0.03 endotoxin unit (EU)/ml [28]. The use of ultrapure dialysis fluid is associated with a reduction in inflammatory markers and an improvement in serum albumin, haemoglobin and ferritin [29].

4. Increasing haemodialysis frequency and length with home haemodialysis

The seminal paper in 1992 by Bernard Charra and his group in Tassin, France, showed hugely impressive survival rates of their haemodialysis patients of 87% at 5 years and 43% at 20 years, which far surpassed matched patients on both European and US registries. All patients received 8 hours of haemodialysis three times per week (LHD). It is likely that the survival association is related to achieving good blood pressure control (antihypertensives were seldom required in the group) through optimized ultrafiltration and the enhanced clearance of uraemic toxins provided by the longer treatment. Their publication sparked interest once again in extended haemodialysis. With the continued increasing demand for renal replacement therapy and limited resources in hospitals, novel ways of providing haemodialysis were required. Home haemodialysis seemed an attractive option and could also accommodate more frequent and extended schedules. The first daily nocturnal haemodialysis programme was set up in Toronto in 1994 [30].

The prescription of home haemodialysis in the United Kingdom remains very variable; however, the most common prescription in 2009 was still 4 hours thrice weekly (51.9% of home HD patients), followed by alternate day dialysis (20.5%), short daily (17.4%) and nocturnal (2.9%) [31]. This is a surprising finding given the benefits of more frequent and extended haemodialysis (which we will now expand on). This does however reflect patient choice and the comfort of both patients and clinicians with a CHD schedule.

4.1. The benefits of extended and more frequent haemodialysis

Several benefits have come to light from more frequent and extended haemodialysis and these will be outlined in this section.

4.1.1. Survival, cardiovascular outcomes and hospitalizations

Observational studies show a significant mortality benefit associated with home haemodialysis, even when adjustments are made for age and comorbidity [32]. These findings are also apparent in studies in Australia and New Zealand [33], which have a higher uptake of home haemodialysis. Figures of 90% survival at 5 years and 45% at 20 years have been quoted [34]. **Figure 1** shows a clear survival advantage to home haemodialysis over both peritoneal dialysis and facility-based HD. These data have to be interpreted with care given the high number of confounders. Patients selected for home haemodialysis are generally younger with a low comorbidity burden. They are usually highly motivated and take an interest in their healthcare.

The frequent haemodialysis network (FHN) trials were setup to give a more definitive answer to the benefits of more frequent and extended haemodialysis [35, 36]. The SDHD arm of the trial randomized 245 patients to either frequent (6 times per week) or conventional haemodialysis and the nocturnal arm randomized 87 patients to either CHD or LDNHD. Two coprimary composite endpoints were used—death or change in LV mass or death or change in physical-health composite score. There was a favourable outcome with regard to both coprimary endpoints for the SDHD trial but not with the LNDHD trial. Looking purely at survival, there was no significant benefit from either trial. With a 12-month follow-up period and the numbers involved with the trials, they were not powered to detect an effect on mortality. The question therefore still remains unanswered as to whether more frequent and extended haemodialysis does have a favourable effect on survival.

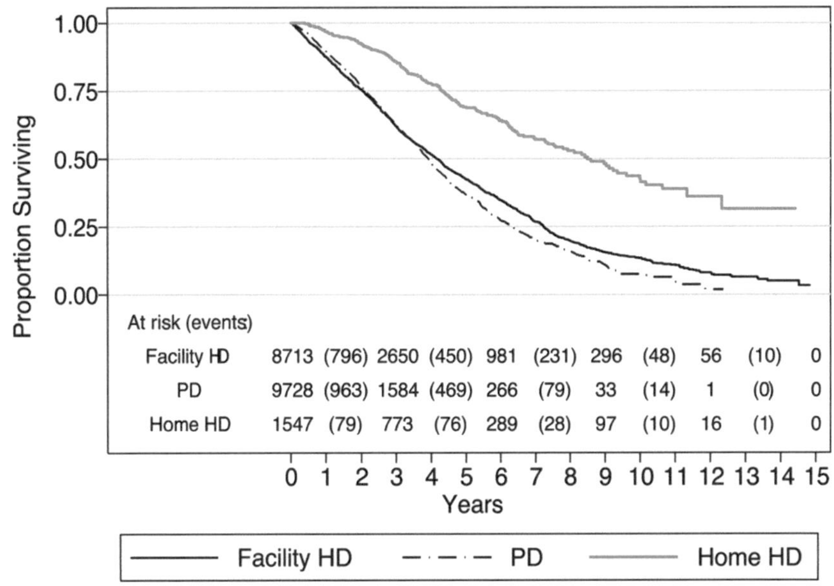

Figure 1. The survival of home HD patients in New Zealand compared with facility HD and peritoneal dialysis (PD). Image adapted from Marshall et al. [35].

There is an associated reduction in cardiovascular-related admissions in converting patients from CHD to LDNHD [37]. There are also fewer cardiovascular-associated hospital admissions associated with SDHD compared with matched CHD; however, all-cause hospitalizations remain unchanged [38]. The FHN studies once again showed no change in the rate of hospitalizations.

4.1.2. *Ultrafiltration and blood pressure control*

There is a strong association between a high ultrafiltration rate (>10 ml/kg/hour) and mortality [39, 40]. Chronic fluid overload contributes to an increased LV mass and congestive cardiac failure [41] and this is likely to be highly significant in terms of cardiovascular morbidity and mortality. Increasing haemodialysis treatment time improves the tolerance of ultrafiltration [42, 43]. There are also many reports of improved blood pressure control both in LNHD and in SDH [44–46] and a regression of left ventricular hypertrophy [47]. It has also been shown that ejection fraction, in those with heart failure, can be improved through more frequent haemodialysis and ultrafiltration [48]. With CHD, it often the case that dry weight is not achieved. Patients that experience hypotension during haemodialysis often have their ultrafiltration stopped, receive saline infusions and thus never achieve their dry weight and in fact can exacerbate the situation further. Extended dialysis allows much lower ultrafiltration rates and thus less haemodynamic disturbance. It is likely the effect that extended dialysis has on blood pressure goes beyond the optimization of volume status. When compared to patients on CHD, some patients with a high extracellular volume (measured by bioimpedance) but on extended haemodialysis achieve normotension [49]. A theory put forward for this phenomenon is that extended haemodialysis may lead to efficient removal of vasoactive factors that contribute to hypertension.

4.1.3. *Small molecule clearance*

Increasing haemodialysis frequency provides more efficient clearance of small MW molecules. It provides a lower peak urea, lower mean urea and less fluctuation [50]. This provides a lower time-averaged concentration (TAC). Looking purely at K_t/V would, however, be misleading as this would remain the same despite the enhanced clearance.

4.1.4. *Phosphate balance*

There is a clear association between raised serum phosphate and adverse cardiovascular outcomes in patients with CKD [51, 52]. Conventional haemodialysis does provide sufficient phosphate removal for western diets, and as a result, there is a net phosphate gain [53]. As a result of this, multiple phosphate binder tablets are often required to reduce the absorption of phosphate from the gut. On average, haemodialysis patients have an average pill burden of 19 pills per day and many of these are phosphate binders [54]. A higher pill burden in this setting is associated with lower quality of life scores [54].

Phosphate removal on haemodialysis has been found to be time dependent [55] and thus is significantly enhanced in NHD. Phosphate removal is also increased by SDHD but not to the same extent as NHD [56]. In LNDHD, many patients will discontinue their phosphate binders [57] and some require supplementation that can be added to the dialysate [58].

4.1.5. *Anaemia*

Reports are mixed when it comes to more frequent haemodialysis and anaemia management. Reduced erythropoietin doses have been reported when patients switch to SDHD from CHD [59] and in NHD [60]. One of the theories put forward for this change is the control of inflammation and reduction in IL-6 levels which improve erythropoietin responsiveness [61]. The exact effect that more frequent or extended dialysis has on anaemia, however, is still unclear. Again both FHN studies showed no effect on erythropoietin dose.

4.1.6. *Quality-of-life measures and carer burden*

Home haemodialysis allows patients the independence to fit their dialysis treatment around their lifestyles. One may expect this to bring significantly improvements to quality of life; however, this may be offset by the burden of having to perform the treatment so frequently, which can lead to burnout or the increased burden on carers. While there are many reports of improvements in quality-of-life measures from switching to NHD [62] or SDHD [63], some show only small improvements in kidney-specific measure of quality of life [64], while others show no difference. Larger studies have shown a reduction in depressive symptoms related to increased dialysis frequency [65].

Data from the recent FHN daily trial showed a significant increase in quality-of-life score in the SDHD group [35] with no specific benefit from NHD over CHD at home. In the FHN NHD arm, however, both groups had an increase in their quality-of-life score showing the positive effect that the setting of the haemodialysis treatment has on this outcome [36] regardless of prescription. Perceived burden on unpaid carers is high among HD patients [66]; however, the FHN trials did not show a higher perceived burden with either SDHD or LDNHD [67].

The patient-reported experience on both LDNHD and SDHD has been positive in terms of physical, psychological and lifestyle aspects [68]. There is also an associated faster recovery time with home haemodialysis [69]. Once again, it is fair to say once again that the jury is still with regard to whether these treatments truly impact on quality of life. In general, the effect seems to be positive with a paucity of data suggesting a negative impact.

4.1.7. Pregnancy

Intensive dialysis has been used very successfully in pregnancy. A case series from Canada [70] shows a markedly improved live birth rate and duration of pregnancy with a dose response between dialysis and pregnancy outcomes. Women who had >36 hours of dialysis per week had significantly improved live birth rates (85 vs. 45% in those who had <20 hours of dialysis per week), which again demonstrates and gives strength to high-dose dialysis.

4.2. Disadvantages of more frequent and home haemodialysis

While there are many advantages of home haemodialysis, the treatment is not suitable for all patients and it is not a treatment without disadvantages. Although exceedingly rare, there is always the possibility that human error can occur resulting in significant blood loss through a variety of mechanisms. There are reports of patient deaths from exsanguination while on home haemodialysis [71]. The sophistication of safety mechanisms is continually improving to make this event less likely with blood leak detectors, pressure monitoring and line disconnect detectors featuring on newer machines.

A clear finding from the FHN trial was an increase in interventions needed for vascular access with 47% of the frequent dialysis group requiring intervention compared with 29% in the CHD group. Interventions to fistulas were required much more often than in catheters. This was not an entirely surprising finding given the considerably increased use of vascular access form more frequent haemodialysis. A solution to this could be the use of a buttonhole technique for fistula cannulation or using single-needle haemodialysis to reduce the number of needling events. The evidence, however, is not there to support this practice and a systematic review of buttonhole cannulation in home haemodialysis patients found an increase in infectious events, an increase in staff support required and no reduction in surgical interventions compared with the "rope ladder" technique [72]. The FHN nocturnal trial used single-needle haemodialysis, and despite this, there was still a trend towards increased vascular interventions in this group.

Finally, globally, the uptake of extended higher frequency haemodialysis remains low, despite a range of benefits and favourable health economics. There can be major patient and clinical factors driving modality uptake. A key determinant, however, is patient motivation and choice. Extended time or frequency on home HD may add to patient and carer burden and is therefore often perceived as a barrier limiting its uptake.

5. Haemodiafiltration

Haemofiltration allows clearance of solutes of up to 20 kDa through the process of convection as previously described. Large volumes of replacement fluid are required for the treatment, and this can be administered either before the filter (pre-dilution) or after the filter (post-dilution). Newer technology also allows a mix of pre- and post-dilution or mid-dilution in an attempt to gain the advantages of both pre- and post-dilution (largely the anticoagulant requirement) [73].

Conventional HDF provides enhanced B2M clearance compared with HD [74]. It is associated with a reduction in pro-inflammatory cytokines such as IL-6 and TNF-α [75] and reduced episodes of hypotension during treatment [76]. There does not appear to be a benefit in terms of left ventricular mass, pulse wave velocity or ejection fraction [77]. This could be due to achieving low substitution volumes or large interdialytic fluid shifts induced by conventional thrice-weekly schedule.

There have been three recent large prospective clinical trials, which have compared HDF with high-flux HD with contrasting results. The ESHOL study [78], a Spanish study, showed promising results with a 30% lower all-cause mortality, a 33% lower cardiovascular mortality and 55% lower infection-related mortality compared with haemodialysis. A Dutch study [79] showed no difference in outcome between HDF and HD and a Turkish [80] study drew the same conclusion. Looking back at these studies, the ESHOL study achieved the highest convective volumes (22.9–23.9 l per session) and *post hoc* analyses of the Turkish and Dutch study also show an association between high convection volume and a survival benefit.

In order to provide HDF with high convection volumes, large volumes of sterile replacement fluid are required (>15 l), which would not be practical with pre-packaged solutions. Instead of online preparation of fluid, which is the most practical solution, HDF uses an additional 50–80 l of water per session [81] (with a typical haemodialysis session using around 500 l of mains water to generate dialysate [82]). Ultrapure dialysate must be generated by the machine to the standards previously described.

5.1. Adding HDF in the home setting

There appears to be a benefit from high convective volume haemodiafiltration. The biggest determinants to achieving a high convective volume are treatment time and blood flow [83].

A blood flow between 360 and 500 ml/min is required to achieve the necessary transmembrane pressure [84]. A well-functioning vascular access would therefore also be required. Although there are reports of achieving a convective volume of >20 l with a haemodialysis catheter, a well-functioning AV fistula would allow higher blood flows [84].

Given that treatment time is clearly an important factor in achieving the dose of HDF associated with improved outcomes, the home setting is an ideal place to deliver the treatment. Vascular access would not be a barrier and combining frequent haemodialysis with a convective treatment should maximize middle molecule clearance. Switching patients from a conventional HDF schedule to a short daily schedule has been reported to result in a higher removal of middle and large molecules, a reduction in phosphate binders, the disappearance of post-dialysis fatigue, an improvement in nutritional status as well as a 30% reduction in left ventricular mass [85]. The improvements in switching to more frequent OL-HDF are outlined in **Table 1**.

	Baseline	Month 3	Month 6
spK_t/V	2.30 ± 0.20	1.13 ± 0.15[b]	1.11 ± 0.11[b]
eK_t/V	1.96 ± 0.17	0.90 ± 0.12[b]	0.88 ± 0.08[b]
URR %	84.3 ± 2.5	64.2 ± 5.3[b]	63.3 ± 4.2[b]
Weekly spK_t/V	6.90 ± 0.59	6.78 ± 0.91	6.67 ± 0.64
Weekly eK_t/V	5.88 ± 0.52	5.39 ± 0.75[a]	5.30 ± 0.50[a]
EKR *mL/min*	19.2 ± 0.5	24.2 ± 2.6[b]	23.8 ± 1.9[b]
stdK_t/V	2.62 ± 0.1	3.87 ± 0.3[b]	3.86 ± 0.2[b]
Weekly URR %	253 ± 7.5	385 ± 32[b]	380 ± 25[b]

a: $P<0.05$;

b: $P<0.01$ with respect to baseline value.

Adapted from Maduell et al. [85].

Abbreviations: URR, urea reduction ratio; spK_t/V, single-pool K_t/V; eK_t/V, equilibrated K_t/V; stdK_t/V, standard K_t/V; TAC, time average concentration; TAD, time average deviation; ERK, equivalent renal urea clearance.

Table 1. Change from three times a week on-line haemodiafiltration (OL-HDF) to short daily on-line haemodiafiltration (D-OL-HDF): comparison of urea kinetics during the two study periods.

While the technology to provide HDF in the home setting exists, it is not widely used at present and there is very little published literature about HDF as a home therapy. Until recently, there have not been haemodialysis machines specifically manufactured for the home market. As a result, patients have been trained on the machines used in the main dialysis unit. Using the same technology both in the home and in the main dialysis unit makes the logistics of maintenance much easier. The health care team, including the technicians, are often more comfortable and experienced using and providing support for a single machine. As technology has developed and haemodialysis machines have become more advanced, it is important that more user-friendly technology, specifically for the home market, is developed. This will allow further uptake and expansion of home dialysis programmes.

The ideal home HD machine has been described [86] as one which is fast and easy to setup, allows a range of prescriptions (such as short daily and nocturnal), teaches and interacts with the patient and allows the patient to deliver intravenous fluid at the push of a button. The description suggests the ability of the machine to re-use blood sets and dialysers, prepare all fluids to a standard beyond ultrapure and have the ability to provide HDF. There are many machines in development and it is likely that this "ideal machine" will be in existence in the near future. There is the potential for HDF machines to be complex given the choice in pre-dilution, post-dilution and mixed dilution and the blood and dialysate flow. Technology should strike a balance, remaining simple for safe use with minimal margin for error and fast training times but also allow some flexibility to tailor treatment.

As previously described, providing a high water quality is of great importance given the high volume that is infused into the patient. The body of evidence to support the use of ultrapure water really lies in convective treatments, and thus, an essential requirement for any home HDF programme will be the production of ultrapure dialysate. Water may contain both chemical and microbiological contaminants, and in the home setting, this is likely to vary considerably depending on the local feed water. A variety of contaminants can have clinical consequences, such as chloramines, leading to haemolytic anaemia [87], calcium and magnesium contributing to a "hard water syndrome" [88] and nitrates [89], zinc [90] and fluorides [91] have all been documented to have potential clinical effects. After initial assessment of the feed water and the subsequent installation of the filters and water softeners, a surveillance programme for chemical contaminants, endotoxins and bacteria is important. This logistics of such a programme needs to be considered as the sampling protocol, laboratory protocols and the transport and storage of samples must all be carefully planned.

Microbiological contamination can still theoretically occur. Reverse osmosis units filter out substances with a molecular weight > 200 kDa and thus bacterial fragments and small endotoxins can still pass through [92]. Vigilance must be employed for unexplained febrile episodes or signs of chronic inflammation. This would apply to both home haemodialysis and haemodiafiltration.

Portability is an important factor for dialysis patients. Peritoneal dialysis has provided a treatment that can be carried out virtually anywhere making the treatment appealing for patients who work or need to travel. To date, the quantity of water and the size of the water treatment devices has limited the portability of haemodialysis. Increasingly, there are haemodialysis machines that allow portability by utilizing sorbent technology to purify water and thus reduce water requirements [93]. With the high convective volumes required for adequate HDF, water requirements remain high and thus limit portability. Developments in this area are needed allow to make HDF a more appealing home treatment for patients. Water use must be minimized and where possible, water should be recycled. Water rejected from reverse osmosis units can be recycled and used elsewhere in the home or dialysis unit and this is being increasingly utilized [82].

Anticoagulation must be a major consideration for any extracorporeal dialysis therapy. Many patients on home haemodialysis manage well with the administration anticoagulation, and unfractionated heparin and low molecular weight heparin are in common use. These strategies can also be used in HDF and should not pose a barrier to home HDF use. HDF may allow dialysis without anticoagulation through the use of pre-dilution HDF. This may be particularly helpful in patients with prolonged bleeding or intolerances to anticoagulation.

Today's dialysis technology enables HDF to be delivered in the home setting safely with the production of ultra-pure dialysate and detection of venous dislodgement. There is a growing experience of centres using this technology [94] with a positive experience. Further details on optimal heparinization regimes, water quality variability and its surveillance in home HDF are necessary to define best clinical practice. It is likely that new technology coupled with increasing HDF uptake in dialysis centres will lead on to increasing use of HDF at home.

5.2. Economic impact of HD and HDF

Haemodialysis treatment in general is very costly, and in the United Kingdom, 1–2% of the National Health Service budget is spent on renal care with only 0.05% with ESRF [95]. After consumables, a large proportion of the cost is made up of direct nursing care and transportation [96] (both of which are considerably less in home haemodialysis). Home haemodialysis has been estimated to cost over a third less than hospital-based haemodialysis in the United Kingdom [96] and frequent home haemodialysis has been shown to offer a cost saving in both Canada and Australia too [97].

In addition to the reduced transport and nursing costs, savings are also offered from a reduction in hospital admissions [37] and a reduction in medication costs (particularly phosphate binders) [98].

The initial setup costs of home haemodialysis are high due to the cost of training, the equipment and installation. These initial costs are usually paid back by 14 months after which savings occur [99], making home haemodialysis an attractive option not only from the clinical benefits but also from the cost-saving aspect.

Costs of high-flux dialysers have also reduced considerably over time and high-flux haemodialysis is now the common standard care. A UK Study looked at the costs of 34 patients switching to OL-HDF and 44 who remained on high-flux HD. The cost of the treatment was either more expensive or cheaper depending on the choice of blood lines. There was a cost saving in the OL-HDF group in terms of phosphate binders. Lebourg et al. [81] looked at >28,000 dialysis treatments in a single centre and once again HDF was found to be either cheaper or more costly (-€1.29 to +€4.58 per session) depending on treatment variables selected. It is clear that from a cost perspective, there is little difference between HDF and high-flux HD.

6. Conclusion

Home haemodialysis provides a convenient and clinically effective way of providing both frequent and extended haemodialysis treatment. Although the hard outcome data for survival from prospective randomized trials are lacking, it is unlikely that a larger, adequately powered trial with sufficient follow-up time will be feasible and the answer may need to come from registry data. It is also time to look beyond urea clearance and towards markers, such as convective volume and β-trace protein, as this may pave the way to further improve haemodialysis care in the future.

However, it is clear that there are a number of clinical benefits from more frequent and extended haemodialysis and aside from this, home haemodialysis is a treatment preferred by many patients if choices are given [100] and a treatment that is associated with an increased satisfaction [101].

HDF is also a feasible treatment in the home setting and is already in use. There is growing evidence from randomized trials that dialysis patient outcomes may be improved by high-frequency HD and by using HDF with high convective volumes. Combining increased frequency HD with convective treatment would give patients the benefits of both small and middle MW clearance without additional patient burden or cost implications. This may pave the way to further improved patient outcomes; however, further randomized clinical studies will be needed for a more definitive answer.

Author details

Sandip Mitra and Kunaal Kharbanda*

*Address all correspondence to: k.kharbanda@nhs.net

Department of Nephrology, Central Manchester Foundation Trust, Manchester Academy of Health Sciences Centre (MAHSC), Manchester, United Kingdom

References

[1] Paskalev DN. Georg Haas (1886–1971): the forgotten hemodialysis pioneer. Dial Transplant. 2001; 30(12):828.

[2] Chapter 1: incidence, prevalence, patient characteristics, and treatment modalities. Am J Kidney Dis. Elsevier; 2016 Mar 1;67(3):S139–58.

[3] Rao A, Casula A, Castledine C. UK renal registry 17th annual report: chapter 2 UK renal replacement therapy prevalence in 2013: national and centre-specific analyses. Nephron. Karger Publishers; 2015;129 Suppl 1(s1):31–56.

[4] Steenkamp R, Rao A, Roderick P. UK renal registry 17th annual report: chapter 5 survival and cause of death in UK adult patients on renal replacement therapy in 2013: national and centre-specific analyses. Nephron. Karger Publishers; 2015;129(s1):99–129.

[5] Thomson GE, Waterhouse K, McDonald HP, Friedman EA. Hemodialysis for chronic renal failure. Clinical observations. Arch Intern Med. 1967 Aug;120(2):153–67.

[6] Shaldon S, Silva H, Rosen SM. Technique of refrigerated coil preservation haemodialysis with femoral venous catheterization. Br Med J. 1964 Aug 15;2(5406):411–3.

[7] Lowrie EG, Laird NM, Parker TF, Sargent JA. Effect of the hemodialysis prescription of patient morbidity: report from the National Cooperative Dialysis Study. N Engl J Med. 1981 Nov 12;305(20):1176–81.

[8] Keshaviah P. Urea kinetic and middle molecule approaches to assessing the adequacy of hemodialysis and CAPD. Kidney Int Suppl. 1993 Feb;40:S28–38.

[9] Lowrie EG, Zhu X, Lew NL. Primary associates of mortality among dialysis patients: trends and reassessment of Kt/V and urea reduction ratio as outcome-based measures of dialysis dose. Am J Kidney Dis.; 1998 Dec;32(6):S16–31.

[10] Foley RN, Gilbertson DT, Murray T, Collins AJ. Long interdialytic interval and mortality among patients receiving hemodialysis. N Engl J Med. 2011 Sep 22;365(12): 1099–107.

[11] Eckardt K-U, Gillespie IA, Kronenberg F, Richards S, Stenvinkel P, Anker SD, et al. High cardiovascular event rates occur within the first weeks of starting hemodialysis. Kidney Int. 2015 Apr 29;88(5):1117–25.

[12] Henderson LW, Besarab A, Michaels A, Bluemle LW. Blood purification by ultrafiltration and fluid replacement (diafiltration). Hemodial Int. 2004 Jan 1;8(1):10–8.

[13] Dhondt A, Vanholder R, Van Biesen W, Lameire N. The removal of uremic toxins. Kidney Int Suppl. 2000 Aug;76:S47–59.

[14] Leypoldt JK, Cheung AK, Carroll CE, Stannard DC, Pereira BJ, Agodoa LY, et al. Effect of dialysis membranes and middle molecule removal on chronic hemodialysis patient survival. Am J Kidney Dis. 1999 Feb;33(2):349–55.

[15] Gejyo F, Yamada T, Odani S, Nakagawa Y, Arakawa M, Kunitomo T, et al. A new form of amyloid protein associated with chronic hemodialysis was identified as beta 2-microglobulin. Biochem Biophys Res Commun. 1985 Jun 28;129(3):701–6.

[16] Lindström V, Grubb A, Alquist Hegbrant M, Christensson A. Different elimination patterns of beta-trace protein, beta2-microglobulin and cystatin C in haemodialysis, haemodiafiltration and haemofiltration. Scand J Clin Lab Invest. 2008;68(8):685–91.

[17] Shafi T, Parekh RS, Jaar BG, Plantinga LC, Oberai PC, Eckfeldt JH, et al. Serum β-trace protein and risk of mortality in incident hemodialysis patients. Clin J Am Soc Nephrol. 2012 Sep;7(9):1435–45.

[18] Craddock PR, Fehr J, Dalmasso AP, Brighan KL, Jacob HS. Hemodialysis leukopenia. Pulmonary vascular leukostasis resulting from complement activation by dialyzer cellophane membranes. J Clin Invest. 1977 May;59(5):879–88.

[19] Simon P, Potier J, Thebaud HE. Risk factors for acute hypersensitivity reactions in hemodialysis. Nephrologie. 1996;17(3):163–70.

[20] Eknoyan G, Beck GJ, Cheung AK, Daugirdas JT, Greene T, Kusek JW, et al. Effect of dialysis dose and membrane flux in maintenance hemodialysis. N Engl J Med. 2002;347(25):2010–9.

[21] Locatelli F, Mastrangelo F, Redaelli B, Ronco C, Marcelli D, La Greca G, et al. Effects of different membranes and dialysis technologies on patient treatment tolerance and nutritional parameters. The Italian Cooperative Dialysis Study Group. Kidney Int. 1996 Oct;50(4):1293–302.

[22] Küchle C, Fricke H, Held E, Schiffl H. High-flux hemodialysis postpones clinical manifestation of dialysis-related amyloidosis. Am J Nephrol. 1996;16(6):484–8.

[23] Bloembergen WE, Hakim RM, Stannard DC, Held PJ, Wolfe RA, Agodoa LY, et al. Relationship of dialysis membrane and cause-specific mortality. Am J Kidney Dis. 1999 Jan;33(1):1–10.

[24] Koda Y, Nishi S, Miyazaki S, Haginoshita S, Sakurabayashi T, Suzuki M, et al. Switch from conventional to high-flux membrane reduces the risk of carpal tunnel syndrome and mortality of hemodialysis patients. Kidney Int. 1997 Oct;52(4):1096–101.

[25] Cheung AK, Levin NW, Greene T, Agodoa L, Bailey J, Beck G, et al. Effects of high-flux hemodialysis on clinical outcomes: results of the HEMO study. J Am Soc Nephrol. 2003 Dec;14(12):3251–63.

[26] Locatelli F, Martin-Malo A, Hannedouche T, Loureiro A, Papadimitriou M, Wizemann V, et al. Effect of membrane permeability on survival of hemodialysis patients. J Am Soc Nephrol. 2009 Feb 25;20(3):645–54.

[27] Tattersall J, Canaud B, Heimbürger O, Pedrini L, Schneditz D, Van Biesen W, et al. High-flux or low-flux dialysis: a position statement following publication of the Membrane Permeability Outcome study. Nephrol Dial Transplant. 2010 Apr 1;25(4): 1230–2.

[28] Glorieux G, Neirynck N, Veys N, Vanholder R. Dialysis water and fluid purity: more than endotoxin. Nephrol Dial Transplant. 2012 Nov;27(11):4010–21.

[29] Rahmati MA, Homel P, Hoenich NA, Levin R, Kaysen GA, Levin NW. The role of improved water quality on inflammatory markers in patients undergoing regular dialysis. Int J Artif Organs. 2004 Aug;27(8):723–7.

[30] Pierratos A, Ouwendyk M, Francoeur R, Vas S, Raj DS, Ecclestone AM, et al. Nocturnal hemodialysis: three-year experience. J Am Soc Nephrol. 1998 May;9(5):859–68.

[31] Gossage-Worrall R, Clift M, lowin J. CEP10061–Buyers' guide: home haemodialysis devices. 2010 Mar 24;1–57.

[32] Woods JD, Port FK, Stannard D, Blagg CR, Held PJ. Comparison of mortality with home hemodialysis and center hemodialysis: a national study. Kidney Int. 1996 Jan 1;49(5): 1464–70.

[33] Marshall MR, HAWLEY CM, Kerr PG, Polkinghorne KR, Marshall RJ, Agar JWM, et al. Home hemodialysis and mortality risk in Australian and New Zealand populations. Am J Kidney Dis. 2011 Nov;58(5):782–93.

[34] Arkouche W, Traeger J, Delawari E, Sibaï-Galland R, Abdullah E, Galland R, et al. Twenty-five years of experience with out-center hemodialysis. Kidney Int. 1999 Dec; 56(6):2269–75.

[35] FHN Trial Group, Chertow GM, Levin NW, Beck GJ, Depner TA, Eggers PW, et al. In-center hemodialysis six times per week versus three times per week. N Engl J Med. 2010 Dec 9;363(24):2287–300.

[36] Rocco MV, Lockridge RS, Beck GJ, Eggers PW, Gassman JJ, Greene T, et al. The effects of frequent nocturnal home hemodialysis: the Frequent Hemodialysis Network Nocturnal Trial. Kidney Int. 2011 Nov;80(10):1080–91.

[37] Bergman A, Fenton SSA, Richardson RMA, Chan CT. Reduction in cardiovascular related hospitalization with nocturnal home hemodialysis. Clin Nephrol. 2008 Jan; 69(1):33–9.

[38] Weinhandl ED, Nieman KM, Gilbertson DT, Collins AJ. Hospitalization in daily home hemodialysis and matched thrice-weekly in-center hemodialysis patients. Am J Kidney Dis. 2015 Jan;65(1):98–108.

[39] Saran R, Bragg-Gresham JL, Levin NW, Twardowski ZJ, Wizemann V, Saito A, et al. Longer treatment time and slower ultrafiltration in hemodialysis: associations with reduced mortality in the DOPPS. Kidney Int. 2006 Apr;69(7):1222–8.

[40] Movilli E, Gaggia P, Zubani R, Camerini C, Vizzardi V, Parrinello G, et al. Association between high ultrafiltration rates and mortality in uraemic patients on regular haemodialysis. A 5-year prospective observational multicentre study. Nephrol Dial Transplant. 2007 Dec;22(12):3547–52.

[41] Parfrey PS. Cardiac disease in dialysis patients: diagnosis, burden of disease, prognosis, risk factors and management. Nephrol Dial Transplant. 2000;15 Suppl 5:58–68.

[42] Brunet P, Saingra Y, Leonetti F, Vacher-Coponat H, Ramananarivo P, Berland Y. Tolerance of haemodialysis: a randomized cross-over trial of 5-h versus 4-h treatment time. Nephrol Dial Transplant. 1996;11 Suppl 8:46–51.

[43] Laurent G, Charra B. The results of an 8 h thrice weekly haemodialysis schedule. Nephrol Dial Transplant. 1998;13 Suppl 6:125–31.

[44] Chan CT, Harvey PJ, Picton P, Pierratos A, Miller JA, Floras JS. Short-term blood pressure, noradrenergic, and vascular effects of nocturnal home hemodialysis. Hypertension. 2003 Nov;42(5):925–31.

[45] Culleton BF, Walsh M, Klarenbach SW, Mortis G, Scott-Douglas N, Quinn RR, et al. Effect of frequent nocturnal hemodialysis vs conventional hemodialysis on left ventricular mass and quality of life: a randomized controlled trial. JAMA. 2007 Sep 19;298(11):1291–9.

[46] Fagugli RM, Pasini P, Pasticci F, Ciao G, Cicconi B, Buoncristiani U. Effects of short daily hemodialysis and extended standard hemodialysis on blood pressure and cardiac hypertrophy: a comparative study. J Nephrol. 2006 Jan;19(1):77–83.

[47] Chan CT, Floras JS, Miller JA, Richardson RMA, Pierratos A. Regression of left ventricular hypertrophy after conversion to nocturnal hemodialysis. Kidney Int. 2002 Jun;61(6):2235–9.

[48] Toz H, Ozkahya M, Ozerkan F, Asci G, Ok E. Improvement in "uremic" cardiomyopathy by persistent ultrafiltration. Hemodial Int. 2007 Jan;11(1):46–50.

[49] Katzarski KS, Charra B, Luik AJ, Nisell J, Divino Filho JC, Leypoldt JK, et al. Fluid state and blood pressure control in patients treated with long and short haemodialysis. Nephrol Dial Transplant. 1999 Feb;14(2):369–75.

[50] Lopot F, Válek A. Quantification of dialysis unphysiology. Nephrol Dial Transplant. 1998;13 Suppl 6:74–8.

[51] Ganesh SK, Stack AG, Levin NW, Hulbert-Shearon T, Port FK. Association of elevated serum PO_4, $CaxPO_4$ product, and parathyroid hormone with cardiac mortality risk in chronic hemodialysis patients. J Am Soc Nephrol. 2001 Oct;12(10):2131–8.

[52] Floege J, Kim J, Ireland E, Chazot C, Drueke T, de Francisco A, et al. Serum iPTH, calcium and phosphate, and the risk of mortality in a European haemodialysis population. Nephrol Dial Transplant. 2011 Jun;26(6):1948–55.

[53] Achinger SG, Ayus JC. The role of daily dialysis in the control of hyperphosphatemia. Kidney Int Suppl. 2005 Jun;67(95):S28–32.

[54] Chiu Y-W, Teitelbaum I, Misra M, de Leon EM, Adzize T, Mehrotra R. Pill burden, adherence, hyperphosphatemia, and quality of life in maintenance dialysis patients. Clin J Am Soc Nephrol. 2009 Jun;4(6):1089–96.

[55] Gutzwiller J-P, Schneditz D, Huber AR, Schindler C, Gutzwiller F, Zehnder CE. Estimating phosphate removal in haemodialysis: an additional tool to quantify dialysis dose. Nephrol Dial Transplant. 2002 Jun;17(6):1037–44.

[56] Al-Hejaili F, Kortas C, Leitch R, Heidenheim AP, Clement L, Nesrallah G, et al. Nocturnal but not short hours quotidian hemodialysis requires an elevated dialysate calcium concentration. J Am Soc Nephrol. 2003 Sep;14(9):2322–8.

[57] Lindsay RM, Alhejaili F, Nesrallah G, Leitch R, Clement L, Heidenheim AP, et al. Calcium and phosphate balance with quotidian hemodialysis. Am J Kidney Dis. 2003 Jul;42(1 Suppl):24–9.

[58] Ebah LM, Akhtar M, Wilde I, Hookway G, Vincent M, Reeves C, et al. Phosphate enrichment of dialysate for use in standard and extended haemodialysis. Blood Purif. 2012;34(1):28–33.

[59] Klarenbach S, Heidenheim AP, Leitch R, Lindsay RM, Daily/Nocturnal Dialysis Study Group. Reduced requirement for erythropoietin with quotidian hemodialysis therapy. ASAIO J. 2002 Jan;48(1):57–61.

[60] Poon CKY, Tang H-L, Wong JHS, Law W-P, Lam C-M, Yim K-F, et al. Effect of alternate night nocturnal home hemodialysis on anemia control in patients with end-stage renal disease. Hemodial Int. 2015 Apr;19(2):235–41.

[61] Yuen D, Richardson RMA, Fenton SSA, McGrath-Chong ME, Chan CT. Quotidian nocturnal hemodialysis improves cytokine profile and enhances erythropoietin responsiveness. ASAIO J. 2005 May;51(3):236–41.

[62] McPhatter LL, Lockridge RS, Albert J, Anderson H, Craft V, Jennings FM, et al. Nightly home hemodialysis: improvement in nutrition and quality of life. Adv Ren Replace Ther. 1999 Oct;6(4):358–65.

[63] Heidenheim AP, Muirhead N, Moist L, Lindsay RM. Patient quality of life on quotidian hemodialysis. Am J Kidney Dis. 2003 Jul;42:36–41.

[64] Manns BJ, Walsh MW, Culleton BF, Hemmelgarn B, Tonelli M, Schorr M, et al. Nocturnal hemodialysis does not improve overall measures of quality of life compared to conventional hemodialysis. Kidney Int. 2009 Mar;75(5):542–9.

[65] Jaber BL, Lee Y, Collins AJ, Hull AR, Kraus MA, McCarthy J, et al. Effect of daily hemodialysis on depressive symptoms and postdialysis recovery time: interim report from the FREEDOM (Following Rehabilitation, Economics and Everyday-Dialysis Outcome Measurements) Study. Am J Kidney Dis. 2010 Sep;56(3):531–9.

[66] Suri RS, Larive B, Garg AX, Hall YN, Pierratos A, Chertow GM, et al. Burden on caregivers as perceived by hemodialysis patients in the Frequent Hemodialysis Network (FHN) trials. Nephrol Dial Transplant. 2011 Jul;26(7):2316–22.

[67] Suri RS, Larive B, Hall Y, Kimmel PL, Kliger AS, Levin N, et al. Effects of frequent hemodialysis on perceived caregiver burden in the frequent hemodialysis network trials. Clin J Am Soc Nephrol. 2014 May 7;9(5):936–42.

[68] Xi W, Singh PM, Harwood L, Lindsay R, Suri R, Brown JB, et al. Patient experiences and preferences on short daily and nocturnal home hemodialysis. Hemodial Int. 2013 Apr 1;17(2):201–7.

[69] Jayanti A, Foden P, Morris J, Brenchley P, Mitra S. Time to recovery from haemodialysis – location, intensity and beyond. Nephrology. 2015 Dec;:n/a–n/a.

[70] Hladunewich MA, Hou S, Odutayo A, Cornelis T, Pierratos A, Goldstein M, et al. Intensive hemodialysis associates with improved pregnancy outcomes: a Canadian and United States cohort comparison. J Am Soc Nephrol. 2014 May;25(5):1103–9.

[71] Allcock K, Jagannathan B, Hood CJ, Marshall MR. Exsanguination of a home hemodialysis patient as a result of misconnected blood-lines during the wash back procedure: a case report. BMC Nephrol. 2012;13(1):28.

[72] Muir CA, Kotwal SS, Hawley CM, Polkinghorne K, Gallagher MP, Snelling P, et al. Buttonhole cannulation and clinical outcomes in a home hemodialysis cohort and systematic review. Clin J Am Soc Nephrol. 2014 Jan;9(1):110–9.

[73] Feliciani A, Riva MA, Zerbi S, Ruggiero P, Plati AR, Cozzi G, et al. New strategies in haemodiafiltration (HDF): prospective comparative analysis between on-line mixed HDF and mid-dilution HDF. Nephrol Dial Transplant. 2007 Jun;22(6):1672–9.

[74] Tattersall J. Clearance of beta-2-microglobulin and middle molecules in haemodiafiltration. Contrib Nephrol. 2007;158:201–9.

[75] Guth HJ, Gruska S, Kraatz G. On-line production of ultrapure substitution fluid reduces TNF-alpha- and IL-6 release in patients on hemodiafiltration therapy. Int J Artif Organs. 2003 Mar;26(3):181–7.

[76] Vilar E, Fry AC, Wellsted D, Tattersall JE, Greenwood RN, Farrington K. Long-term outcomes in online hemodiafiltration and high-flux hemodialysis: a comparative analysis. Clin J Am Soc Nephrol. 2009 Dec;4(12):1944–53.

[77] Mostovaya IM, Bots ML, van den Dorpel MA, Grooteman MPC, Kamp O, Lévesque R, et al. A randomized trial of hemodiafiltration and change in cardiovascular parameters. Clin J Am Soc Nephrol. 2014 Mar;9(3):520–6.

[78] Maduell F, Moreso F, Pons M, Ramos R, Mora-Macià J, Carreras J, et al. High-efficiency postdilution online hemodiafiltration reduces all-cause mortality in hemodialysis patients. J Am Soc Nephrol. 2013 Feb;24(3):487–97.

[79] Grooteman MPC, van den Dorpel MA, Bots ML, Penne EL, van der Weerd NC, Mazairac AHA, et al. Effect of online hemodiafiltration on all-cause mortality and cardiovascular outcomes. J Am Soc Nephrol. 2012 Jun;23(6):1087–96.

[80] Ok E, Asci G, Toz H, Ok ES, Kircelli F, Yilmaz M, et al. Mortality and cardiovascular events in online haemodiafiltration (OL-HDF) compared with high-flux dialysis: results from the Turkish OL-HDF Study. Nephrol Dial Transplant. 2013 Jan;28(1):192–202.

[81] Lebourg L, Amato S, Toledano D, Petitclerc T, Créput C. Online hemodiafiltration: is it really more expensive?. Nephrol Ther. 2013 Jul;9(4):209–14.

[82] Agar JWM. Reusing and recycling dialysis reverse osmosis system reject water. Kidney Int. 2015 Oct;88(4):653–7.

[83] Penne EL, van der Weerd NC, Bots ML, van den Dorpel MA, Grooteman MPC, Lévesque R, et al. Patient- and treatment-related determinants of convective volume in post-dilution haemodiafiltration in clinical practice. Nephrol Dial Transplant. 2009 Nov;24(11):3493–9.

[84] Maduell F. Optimizing the prescription of hemodiafiltration. Contrib Nephrol. 2007;158:225–31.

[85] Maduell F, Navarro V, Torregrosa E, Rius A, Dicenta F, Cruz MC, et al. Change from three times a week on-line hemodiafiltration to short daily on-line hemodiafiltration. Kidney Int. 2003 Jan 1;64(1):305–13.

[86] Kjellstrand CM, Kjellstrand P. The ideal home hemodialysis machine. Hemodial Int. 2008 Jul;12 Suppl 1(s1):S33–9.

[87] Kitching AR, Ritchie D, Wong JK, May A, Hatfield PJ. Chloramine-induced hemolysis associated with neurological symptoms in a home hemodialysis patient. Clin Nephrol. 2001 Mar;55(3):259–60.

[88] Freeman RM, Lawton RL, Chamberlain MA. Hard-water syndrome. N Engl J Med. 1967 May 18;276(20):1113–8.

[89] Carlson DJ, Shapiro FL. Methemoglobinemia from well water nitrates: a complication of home dialysis. Ann Intern Med. 1970 Nov;73(5):757–9.

[90] Gallery ED, Blomfield J, Dixon SR. Acute zinc toxicity in haemodialysis. Br Med J. 1972 Nov 11;4(5836):331–3.

[91] Arnow PM. An outbreak of fatal fluoride intoxication in a long-term hemodialysis unit. Ann Intern Med. 1994 Sep 1;121(5):339–44.

[92] Schindler R, Beck W, Deppisch R, Aussieker M, Wilde A, Göhl H, et al. Short bacterial DNA fragments: detection in dialysate and induction of cytokines. J Am Soc Nephrol. 2004 Dec;15(12):3207–14.

http://dx.doi.org/10.5772/64095

[93] AGAR JW. Review: understanding sorbent dialysis systems. Nephrology. 2010 Mar 19;15(4):406–11.

[94] Walter C. Home haemodiafiltration an optimal treatment. Poster session at Renal Society of Australasia Annual Conference. 2015 Jun 15–17; Perth, Australia.

[95] UK Department of Health (DH). National Service Framework (NSF) renal services part one: dialysis and transplantation. 2004 Jan 8;1–60. Available at: https://www.gov.uk/government/uploads/system/uploads/attachment_data/file/199001/National_Service_Framework_for_Renal_Services_Part_One_-_Dialysis_and_Transplantation.pdf.

[96] Baboolal K, McEwan P, Sondhi S, Spiewanowski P, Wechowski J, Wilson K. The cost of renal dialysis in a UK setting – a multicentre study. Nephrol Dial Transplant. 2008 Jun;23(6):1982–9.

[97] Komenda P, Gavaghan MB, Garfield SS, Poret AW, Sood MM. An economic assessment model for in-center, conventional home, and more frequent home hemodialysis. Kidney Int. 2011 Oct 12;81(3):307–13.

[98] Klarenbach S, Tonelli M, Pauly R, Walsh M, Culleton B, So H, et al. Economic evaluation of frequent home nocturnal hemodialysis based on a randomized controlled trial. J Am Soc Nephrol. 2014 Mar;25(3):587–94.

[99] Delano BG, Feinroth MV, Feinroth M, Friedman EA. Home and medical center hemodialysis. Dollar comparison and payback period. JAMA. 1981 Jul 17;246(3):230–2.

[100] Keating PT, Walsh M, Ribic CM, Brimble KS. The impact of patient preference on dialysis modality and hemodialysis vascular access. BMC Nephrol. 2014 Feb 22;15(1):1.

[101] Fadem SZ, Walker DR, Abbott G, Friedman AL, Goldman R, Sexton S, et al. Satisfaction with renal replacement therapy and education: the American Association of Kidney Patients survey. Clin J Am Soc Nephrol. 2011 Mar;6(3):605–12.

Chapter 8

Quality of Life on Online Hemodiafiltration (HDF)

Samir H. Almueilo

Additional information is available at the end of the chapter

http://dx.doi.org/10.5772/64591

Abstract

Online hemodiafiltration (OL-HDF) as a renal replacement therapy is gaining momentum due to the perceived added benefit from enhanced clearance of potentially harmful middle molecules. Favorable effect of OL-HDF on all-cause mortality and cardiovascular mortality and morbidity has been suggested by some clinical trials. Health-related quality of life (HRQOL) is an important component of hemodialysis patients' care. HRQOL is of interest to both health care providers and patients. Improved quality of life in hemodialysis patients has been associated with improved outcome in terms of reduced rate of hospitalization and mortality. Data on HRQOL in end-stage renal disease (ESRD) patients under OL-HDF is scarce and of marginal quality. In this review, we will try to summarize the available evidence on this subject.

Keywords: Quality of life, Health-related quality of life, Online hemodiafiltration, Hemodiafiltration, End-stage renal disease

1. Introduction

End-stage renal disease (ESRD) is characterized by significantly increase rate of mortality and morbidity. Survival of patients with end-stage renal disease is substantially decreased compared to counterparts without renal failure. It is estimated that 10–20 % of dialysis patients die annually [1]. Historically, in patients with ESRD, survival has been commonly utilized as a measure of outcome, as both health care providers and patients are most interested in prolonging life.

Quality of life (QOL) is curtailed in these patients not only due to the physical burden of the disease but also due to its effect on psychological, social interaction, rehabilitation, and employment component of patient life. Renal replacement therapy decreases morbidity related to uremia and improves many of the uremic symptoms such as anorexia, fatigue, and pruritus that have a negative impact on the quality of daily life.

Conventional hemodialysis (HD) is reasonably effective in removing small solutes by way of diffusion across membranes. However, middle molecules which are implicated in adverse outcome are poorly removed by such mechanism. Secondary analysis of the HD trial had suggested that survival may depend on clearance of such middle molecules [2]. Convective therapy is more effective in removing larger toxic middle molecules such as β2-microglobulin. High-volume online hemodiafiltration (OL-HDF) effectively achieves significant clearance of middle molecules. Such treatment has been shown to be beneficial in terms of lower risk of all-cause and cardiovascular mortality when compared to standard hemodialysis. Secondary analysis of initially negative clinical trials also demonstrated decreased mortality in recipients of high-volume OL-HDF [3–7].

Hemodiafiltration (HDF) combines diffusive and convective clearance of uremic solutes. It involves convection of large volume of fluid and infusing in the patient a replacement fluid that is ultrapure, sterile, and free of pyrogens. Utilization of online HDF where replacement fluid is prepared by further purifying dialysate fluid instead of manufacturer-provided solutions made it more practical and cost effective. It is believed that high-volume HDF by increasing clearance of middle molecules could potentially improve symptomatology, reduces morbidity, and may even improve survival [8]. These in turn could result in improved quality of life. Improved quality of life in hemodialysis patients has been associated with improved outcome. Analysis of data using the Kidney Disease Quality of Life Short Form (KDQOL-SFTM) obtained from 10,030 randomly selected hemodialysis patients from the USA, five European countries and Japan in the Dialysis Outcomes and Practice Patterns Study (DOPPS) demonstrated associations between HRQOL and the risk of death and hospitalization. Scores were determined for three components of HRQOL: (1) physical component summary (PCS), (2) mental component summary (MCS), and (3) kidney disease component summary (KDCS). Lower scores for the three major components of HRQOL were strongly associated with higher risk of death and hospitalization in hemodialysis patients, independent of a number of demographic and comorbid factors [9].

Information on quality of life in patients receiving renal replacement therapy in the form of OL-HDF is scarce and inconclusive. The studies often involve small sample size and uses different methods of quantifying HRQOL. In this report, we will attempt to address HRQOL in patients under OL-HDF treatment by way of defining HRQOL, describing the most common instruments used to evaluate HRQOL and presenting brief summaries of clinical studies that investigated HRQOL in individuals receiving convective therapy.

2. What is health-related quality of life (HRQOL)

The concept of HRQOL has been around for many decades. In its constitution, the World Health Organization has defined health as "a state of complete physical, mental and social

http://dx.doi.org/10.5772/64591

well-being and not merely the absence of disease or infirmity" [10]. Quality of life (QOL) is a broad multidimensional concept that usually includes subjective evaluations of both positive and negative aspects of life [11]. It is often defined differently by variable groups and professional societies. This adds to the difficulty of measuring QOL. Health constitutes an important component of QOL assessment. However, other parameters such as employment, education, housing, and family life are important contributors to the overall QOL. Cultural and religious beliefs and values also add to the complexity of assessing quality of life.

The World Health Organization defines QOL as "an individual's perception of their position in life in the context of the culture and value system where they live, and in relation to their goals, expectations, standards, and concerns" [12]. Assessment of quality of life should encompass not only the physical condition but also factors that have an impact on the individual's well-being such as social, economic, emotional, and psychological factors. Quality of life and health are closely related. Each can have a positive or a negative impact on the other depending on condition. Such a relationship is demonstrated by the notion that greater survival is associated with a higher-measured QOL [13, 14].

Assessments of HRQOL have evolved over the years to include aspects of overall quality of life that can be obviously shown to affect physical as well as mental health (MH) [15–17].

On the individual level, this includes physical and mental health perceptions and their correlates including health risks and conditions, functional status, social support, and socioeconomic status. On the community level, HRQOL includes resources, conditions, policies, and practices that influence a population's health perceptions and functional status. The construct of HRQOL enables health agencies to legitimately address broader areas of public health policy in collaboration with a wider circle of health partners, including social service agencies and community planners.

HRQOL questions about perceived physical and mental health and function have become an important component of health surveillance and are generally considered valid indicators of service needs and intervention outcomes. Self-assessed health status also proved to be a more powerful predictor of mortality and morbidity than many objective measures of health [9].

The measurement of QOL should encompass many factors that affect a subject's well-being. It should include not just the physical aspect but also the social, emotional, intellectual, and cultural components that comprise daily life. According to this foundation, we can define an aspect of QOL as being health related. This health-related quality of life (HRQOL) represents the "physical, psychological, and social domains of health that are influenced by a person's experience, beliefs, expectations, and perceptions" [18]. Each of these domains can be measured in two dimensions, objective assessments of functioning status and subjective perceptions of health as reported by the individual. The patient's subjective attitudes and expectations convert that objective assessment into the actual quality of life [10].

Within this context, health is defined as not only the absence of disease and infirmity but also the presence of physical, mental, and social well-being [11].

3. Measuring health-related quality of life

Adequate HRQOL measurement instrument should capture all the effects that disease and its treatment have on the physical, emotional, social, and mental dimensions of an individual [19]. An ideal instrument would be comprehensive, reliable, and of proven validity and would facilitate comparisons between groups of subjects with different illnesses and within the same group receiving different modes of treatment. The extracted HRQOL measures must be converted into a numerical value for proper utilization.

There is no one ideal tool of measuring HRQOL, and therefore, multiple different instruments have been developed.

Most of these instruments use a series of questions to assess quality of life indirectly. These questions are defined as "items." Each item is then given a numerical value, based on a predetermined scale. Most researchers measure each quality-of-life domain separately, by asking specific questions pertaining to its most important components.

HRQOL instruments can be subdivided into categories based on whether the tool is global or domain specific. Three major domains comprise global HRQOL: the physical domain, the social domain, and the psychosocial or mental domain.

Many schemes have been developed to assess QOL in individuals with end-stage renal disease. Here, we will briefly describe the most common tools used in assessing HRQOL in studies involving patients under treatment by OL-HDF.

Domain	Meaning of low score	Meaning of high score	Number of questions
Physical functioning (PF)	Severe limitations in physical activity, including bathing and dressing	Performs vigorous activity without limitations	10
Role-physical (RP)	Limited ability to work because of physical health	Physical health does not limit work or other activities	4
Bodily pain (BP)	Severe limiting pain	No pain or limitations due to pain	2
General health (GH)	Perceives health as poor	Perceives health as excellent	5
Vitality (VT)	Feels tired and worn out all the time	Feels full of pep and energy all the time	4
Social functioning (SF)	Physical and emotional symptoms severely limit normal social activities	No physical or emotional limits to normal social activities	2
Role-emotional (RE)	Emotions limit daily function and work	Emotions do not interfere with daily function or work	3
Mental health (MH)	Feels nervous and depressed all the time	Feels peaceful, happy, and calm all the time	5

Ref. [25].

Table 1. Components of the Short Form-36 (SF-36).

3.1. Kidney Disease Quality of Life (KDQOL) Short Form-36 (SF-36)

The Kidney Disease Quality of Life (KDQOL) instrument is a self-report questionnaire consisting of 134 items [20]. It has the SF-36 as its generic core and is supplemented with items of relevance to the HRQOL of dialysis patients. Disease-specific items assess symptoms/problems, effects of kidney disease on daily life, burden of kidney disease, cognitive function, work status, sexual function, quality of social interaction, and sleep. Included are also items relating to social support, encouragement from dialysis staff, patient satisfaction with care, and a global rating of health. A more practical shorter version, the KDQOL-SF, was developed later in view of the length of the original one. The KDQOL-SF includes the SF-36 supplemented with 43 disease-specific items from the domains identified in the original version [21].

The KDQOL-SF is easy to administer and has been validated and used widely with hemodialysis (HD) patients. KDQOL-SF became the most widely used QOL measure for ESRD patients. It was developed in the USA for dialysis patients and has been translated into several languages, to be used in several studies involving dialysis patients [22–24].

The SF-36 Health Survey can be self-reported or obtained with the help from a health professional in patients unable to complete the survey. The SF-36 contains only 36 items, through which it evaluates eight health concepts of HRQOL. The eight health concepts are physical functioning (ten items), role limitations resulting from physical problems (four items), role limitations caused by emotional or personal problems (three items), social functioning (two items), bodily pain (BP) (two items), energy/fatigue (four items), emotional well-being (five items), and general health (GH) perceptions (five items). In addition, there is one single item that provides an indication of perceived change since 1 year. Two additional components can be calculated from the SF-36, and they are the physical component summary (PCS) and the mental component summary (MCS). A higher score is associated with a more favorable health status. Components of the SF-36 are depicted in **Table 1**.

3.2. The Kidney Disease Questionnaire (KDQ) of Laupacis et al. (Canada) [26]

In 1992, Laupacis developed this tool which is disease-specific designed for use in chronic HD patients. The KDQ consists of 26 items in five dimensions: physical symptoms (six items), fatigue (six items), depression (five items), relationships (six items), and frustration (three items). The physical symptoms dimension of the KDQ is patient specific. The six physical symptoms that are most important to each subject are identified and used to assess that dimension. Patients are asked to identify their specific physical problems, next to questions regarding frustration, depression, and well-being. Patients are asked to grade their complaints on a scale ranging from one (severe) to seven (none). The KDQ is designed for use only in patients with ESRD on HD treatment.

3.3. The Euro Quality of Life Group (EQ-5DTM) questionnaire

The EQ-5DTM measures health-related quality of life in five dimensions: mobility, self-care, usual activities, pain/discomfort, and anxiety/depression. Scores for the five dimensions are converted into preference weights by using country-specific value sets drawn from the general population [27].

This instrument is rather new; therefore, only few country-specific value sets are available.

3.4. The CHOICE Health Experience Questionnaire (CHEQ) [28]

This is a patient-reported measure of HRQOL developed for use in the Choices for Healthy Outcomes in Caring for End-Stage Renal Disease (CHOICE) Study [29]. The authors have defined it as "the value assigned to duration of life as modified by the impairment, functional states, perceptions, and social opportunities that are influenced by disease, injury, or policy." This instrument was developed to evaluate the effectiveness of alternative dialysis prescriptions. It supplements SF-36 survey in measuring HRQOL for patients with ESRD. It is sensitive to differences in dialysis modality and dialysis dose. The selection of HRQOL domains to be utilized was based on literature review, analysis of focus groups, and survey of dialysis providers and patients. In order to arrange domains and items identified, a representative sample of 136 dialysis patients rated each item for frequency and distress. The survey yielded 22 HRQOL domains that included 96 items: eight generic domains in the SF-36 (health perceptions, physical, social, physical and emotional role functions, pain, mental health, and energy), eight additional generic domains (cognitive functioning, sexual functioning, sleep, work, recreation, travel, finances, and general quality of life), and six ESRD-specific domains (diet, freedom, time, body image, dialysis access, and symptoms).

4. Trials on quality of life in HDF

The results of studies on HRQOL in OL-HDF are often inconclusive. The studies used different questionnaires to assess HRQOL which probably explain some of the differences among studies.

Reference	Country	Comparison	Quality-of-life instrument used	Timing of assessment	Study result
Moura et al. [38]	Portugal	Four age quartiles (<56 years, 57–68 years, 69–75 years, >75 years old)	KDQOL-SF version 1.3 for Portuguese patients	One time at baseline	Women >56 years old had decrease in work status, patient satisfaction, and role-physical. Men had decreasing physical functioning, with increasing age. Compared to women, men generally had higher scores in all quartiles on variable combinations of physical functioning and pain, patient's satisfaction, symptoms/problem list, work status, role-physical, emotional

http://dx.doi.org/10.5772/64591

Reference	Country	Comparison	Quality-of-life instrument used	Timing of assessment	Study result
					well-being, work status, energy/fatigue, and quality of social interactions
Karkar et al. [32]	Saudi Arabia	HF-HD and OL-HDF	Modified KDQOL-SF version 1.3	24 months	OL-HDF was associated with improvement in general mood, body energy, dialysis compliance, sexual performance, social activity, and patient's satisfaction
Moura et al. [43]	Portugal	Access type: AVF vs. CVC	KDQOL-SF version 1.3 for Portuguese patients	One time at baseline	Patients with CVC had a decrease in scores of physical functioning, emotional well-being, role emotional, and energy/fatigue domains when compared with those with AVF. Patients with CVC also showed a decline in cognitive function and quality-of-social interaction domains. Nondiabetic patients generally scored better than diabetic patients with similar vascular access
Mazairac et al. [37]	The Netherlands, Canada, and Norway	OL-HDF and LF-HD	KDQOL-SF-36 version 1.3	At baseline and Q 3 months for a median of 2 years	At baseline, mean PCS and MCS were similar in both groups. In both groups, multiple HRQOL domain scores declined over time. Overall health domain improved in HDF patients. A trend to a worse MCS and an improved effect of kidney disease on daily life in patients on HDF
Kantartzi et al. [33]	Greece	LF-HD vs. OL-HDF and HDF (with prepared bags)	IQOLA SF-36 Greek version	Q 3 months for 1 year	OL-HDF and HDF had better score in bodily pain and role limitations due to emotional functioning. There were no differences between the two types of hemodiafiltration
Knezevic et al. [31]	Serbia	OL-HDF vs. HF-HD and LF-HD	KDQOL-SF-36	One time at baseline	No difference in general health domain. Patients on HDF had better score in most of the domains compared with patients on HD, especially compared with low-flux HD patients. No differences between high-flux HD and low-flux HD Age, economic status, dialysis modality, and ischemic heart disease were

Reference	Country	Comparison	Quality-of-life instrument used	Timing of assessment	Study result
					associated with PCS. Age, sex, economic status, dialysis modality, and vascular access are associated with MCS
Stefánsson et al. [40]	Sweden	OL-HDF vs. LF-HD	IQOLA SF-36 (Swedish version) + local questionnaire	60 days	With the exception of a lower score for social functioning with HDF, there was no significant difference in quality of life between HD and HDF
Schiffl [34]	Germany	HF-HD vs. OL-HDF	KDQ	52 weeks	Patients in the two treatment groups had similar perceptions of their quality of life. While on OL-HDF, patients had sustained improvement in physical symptoms. No change of this dimension with the other mode of therapy
Beerenhout et al. [39]	The Netherlands	OL-HF vs. LF-HD	KDQ	At baseline, 6 and 12 months	Physical symptoms improved in the HF group after 6 and 12 months, but not in the HD group. QOL for other aspects (frustration, depression, well-being) did not change in any treatment group
Lin et al. [44]	Taiwan	OL-HDF vs. HF-HD (different combinations)	Patients' score of subjective well-being, work tolerance, and mental alertness	Weekly	Interdialytic symptomatic hypotensive episodes and interdialysis physical well-being and symptoms improved when frequency of HDF is increased to three times per week
Ward et al. [41]	Germany	OL-HDF vs. HF-HD	The Kidney Disease Questionnaire	26 and 52 weeks	Both groups had similar perceptions of their quality of life. Patients' assessment of physical symptoms improved during the course of the study independent of mode of therapy
Verzetti et al. [42]	Italy	AFB vs. BHD in patients with diabetic ESRD	Patients' score of their degree of subjective well-being	Monthly	Subjective report of well-being increased when patients switched from traditional HD to AFB

Abbreviations: AFB, acetate-free biofiltration; AVF, arteriovenous fistula; BHD, bicarbonate hemodialysis; CVC, central venous catheter; HDF, hemodiafiltration; HF, hemofiltration; HF-HD, high-flux hemodialysis; IQOLA, International Quality of Life Assessment; KDQOL, Kidney Disease Quality of Life; KDQ, Kidney Disease Questionnaire; LF-HD, low-flux hemodialysis; MCS, mental component summary; OL-HDF, online hemodiafiltration; OL-HF, online hemofiltration; PCS, physical component summary; SF-36, Short Form-36.

Table 2. Summary of studies assessing QOL in patients treated with convective therapy.

http://dx.doi.org/10.5772/64591

The following is the description of trials that examined HRQOL in patients under treatment of OL-HDF, hemofiltration (HF), and acetate-free biofiltration (AFB) in comparison to low-flux hemodialysis (LF-HD) or high-flux hemodialysis (HF-HD). Summary of these trials is presented in **Table 2**.

4.1. Moura et al.

Moura et al. performed an evaluation of 322 ESRD under OL-HDF from five dialysis units in north Portugal in which patients reported HRQOL utilizing the Kidney Disease Quality of Life Short Form (KDQOL-SF). Patients showed a mean (±SD) of 53.17 % (±15.31 %) in SF-36 total score, 50.17 % (±9.51 %) in the SF-36 mental component summary (MCS), and 49.75 % (±9.44 %) in the SF-36 physical component summary (PCS). Red cell distribution width (RDW), female gender, and diabetes were found as significant predictors of SF-36 total score of HRQOL, which accounts for 12 % of the total explained variance. Patient satisfaction, RDW, body mass index, and gender were identified as predictors for the PCS, which accounts for 22 % of total explained variance. Furthermore, patient satisfaction and dry weight were found as predictors for MCS. These predictors accounted for 28 % of the total explained variance. The authors concluded that the coexistence of diabetes, female gender, and anemia are predictors of HRQOL in patients under OL-HDF and suggest that more attention should be given to these issues in order to improve HRQOL [30]

4.2. Knezevic et al.

Knezevic et al. examined whether hemodialysis modality and membrane flux, independent of membrane biocompatibility, make differences in quality of life in 124 patients from Serbia. The patients were divided, based on therapy, into three groups: online HDF, high-flux hemodialysis, and low-flux hemodialysis. Health-related quality of life was assessed using the Short Form-36 questionnaire combined with special questionnaire, which included demographic and clinically related questions. Health-related quality of life was better in patients on HDF compared with patients on hemodialysis, especially compared with low-flux hemodialysis patients in most of the scales and in both dimensions: physical component scale and mental component scale. There were no differences in Short Form-36 domains between high-flux hemodialysis and low-flux hemodialysis. The conclusion was that HDF has a potential positive influence on quality of life, which is sufficient to justify further research in prospective and longitudinal study design [31].

4.3. Karkar et al.

Karkar et al. investigated the effect of online HDF vs. high-flux hemodialysis (HF-HD) on a patient's health-related satisfaction level. The study involved 72 patients from Saudi Arabia on regular low-flux HD who were randomized to HF randomized to HF-HD and to HDF (n = 36) and followed up for 24 months. Satisfaction level was assessed using modified questionnaires of the Kidney Disease Quality of Life Short Form (KDQOL-SF) version 1.3. The HDF group achieved a higher satisfaction level than the HD group ($P < 0.0001$) with less cramps, itching, joint pain, and stiffness. There was an improvement in general mood, sexual performance, and social activity. The investigators concluded that high-efficiency postdilution online HDF significantly improved patients' satisfaction level and quality of life [32].

4.4. Kantartzi et al.

Kantartzi et al. reported a prospective crossover study involving 24 patients. Each patient received HD, OL-HDF, and HDF with prepared bags of substitution fluid for 3 months, with the dialysis modality subsequently being altered. Quality of life was measured by the Short-Form Health Survey with 36 questions (SF-36), and subscale scores were calculated. There were statistical significant differences in QOL for the total SF-36, bodily pain score, and role limitations due to emotional functioning in favor of online HDF over low-flux HD [33].

4.5. Schiffl

Schiffl studied 76 clinically stable patients on low-flux conventional HD (LF-HD) in a prospective crossover clinical evaluation of high-flux ultrapure hemodialysis (HF-HD) and OL-HDF. They were randomized to HF-HD or OL-HDF (24 months) and switched to the alternative treatment (24 months). Online HDF had a greater clearance of urea, phosphate, and β2-microglobulin. Both OL-HDF and high-flux ultrapure HD significantly improved nutritional status and the response to erythropoietin. Disease-related quality of life was determined after 52 weeks of each study period using the KDQ. The KDQ determines quality of life in five dimensions: physical symptoms, fatigue, depression, relationship with others, and frustration. The patients in the two treatment groups had similar perceptions of their quality of life. However, the patients' assessment of their physical symptoms showed a sustained improvement during treatment with OL-HDF. There was no change of this dimension with the other modes of therapy ($P < 0.05$). None of the other dimensions of the Kidney Disease Questionnaire showed a change during the course of the study [34].

4.6. Mazairac et al.

Mazairac et al. analyzed data of 714 patients from the Convective Transport Study [35, 36] with a median follow-up of 2 years to assess the effect of HDF on quality of life compared with HD in patients with ESRD. Quality of life was assessed with the KDQOL-SF. There were no significant differences in changes of HRQOL over time between patients treated with HD ($n = 358$) or hemofiltration ($n = 356$) [37].

4.7. Moura et al.

Moura et al. evaluated the influence of aging on patients' perception of HRQOL in 305 ESRD patients under OL-HDF. Data about comorbidities, hematological data, iron status, dialysis adequacy, and nutritional and inflammatory markers were collected from patient's records. Quality of life was assessed by using the KDQOL-SF. Analysis of the data showed significant decrease with increasing age in some parameters evaluated by the KDQOL-SF instrument, namely, for work status, physical functioning, and role-physical (RP) [38].

4.8. Beerenhout et al.

Beerenhout et al. examined the effects of LF-HD and predilution online HF (OL-HF) on cardiovascular and nutritional parameters, interdialytic levels of uremic toxins, and quality of life. The KDQ of Laupacis [26] was used for QOL assessment. At 1 year, 27 patients were eligible for analysis (HF, 13 patients; HD, 14 patients). QOL for physical symptoms improved in the HF group (4.2 ± 1.2–5.0 ± 1.1), $P < 0.05$ within the HF group, but not in the HD group (4.0 ± 1–4.4 ± 1.4) [39].

4.9. Stefánsson et al.

Stefánsson et al. performed a prospective, randomized, and patient-blinded crossover study involving 20 patients from Sweden on chronic HD. The patients received either HD for 2 months followed by postdilution HDF for 2 months or in opposite order. Online postdilution HDF was used, and the replacement volume was standardized to 25–30 % of the total blood volume treated. The two treatments were similar with respect to dialysis-related complications, quality of life, and the biomarkers of oxidative stress and inflammation. Interviews for assessment of quality of life were double blinded. Patients answered health-related questions in two separate questionnaires. The first one was the Swedish version of the standardized quality-of-life questionnaire, SF-36. The second one was generated by the study designers and specifically concerned 12 symptoms and health-related conditions occurring during the previous 4 weeks. With the exception of a lower score for social functioning with HDF ($P < 0.05$), there was no significant difference in quality of life between HD and HDF [40].

4.10. Ward et al.

Ward et al. tested the hypothesis that HDF provides better solute removal than HF-HD in a prospective, randomized clinical trial. Twenty-four patients were randomized to online postdilution HDF, and twenty-one patients were allocated to HF-HD for a period of 12 months. Removal of both small (urea and creatinine) and large (β2-microglobulin and complement factor D) solutes was significantly greater for HDF than for HF-HD. Pretreatment plasma β2-microglobulin concentrations decreased with time ($P < 0.001$); however, the decrease was similar for both therapies. The patients' assessment of their quality of life was determined after 26 and 52 weeks of the study. A single interviewer administered the questionnaire to all patients. The patients in both groups had similar perceptions of their quality of life as assessed by the KDQ. The patients' assessment of their physical symptoms showed a significant improvement during the course of the study which was independent of the treatment modality. None of the other dimensions of the KDQ showed a change over the course of the study [41].

4.11. Verzetti et al.

Verzetti et al. performed a study to compare standard bicarbonate hemodialysis (BHD) with acetate-free biofiltration (AFB) in a group of 41 stable diabetic patients on dialysis treatment for 25 ± 22 months. Twenty-four type II and seventeen type I diabetic patients, all requiring insulin therapy, were included and were followed up for 1 year in a 6-month crossover randomized study for both methods. The analysis was carried out on dialysis symptoms, interdialysis symptoms, and nutritional status. On a monthly basis, patients were also required to score their degree of subjective well-being. All the clinical events occurring during the study period, together with the number of hospitalizations and mortality rates, were recorded. AFB significantly reduced dialytic and extra-dialytic symptoms ($P = 0.003$ and 0.001, respectively). Cardiovascular collapses decreased by 43 %, and other dialysis symptoms showed a similar trend (−35 %). The interdialysis symptoms decreased by 28 % and were accompanied by an increase in subjective well-being (39 %) when patients were switched from traditional HD to AFB. Acid-base control was better with AFB ($P = 0.01$), both at the beginning and during the session. In comparison to traditional HD, hypotensive episodes and other dialysis symptoms during AFB decreased by 43 % and 35 %, respectively. Interdialysis symptoms showed the same favorable trend, decreasing by 28 %. Moreover, subjective report of well-being increased by 39 % when the patients switched from traditional HD to AFB. The number of hospital admissions and the mortality rate were lower during the AFB than the BHD period. The authors concluded that AFB allows better control of some metabolic aspects, reduces intra- and extra-dialysis symptoms, and improves patient QOL [42].

4.12. Moura et al.

Moura et al. examined the effect of vascular access type (arteriovenous fistula (AVF) vs. central venous catheter (CVC)) on patients reported HRQOL in 322 ESRD under OL-HDF. Arteriovenous fistula (AVF) was used by 252 patients (78.3 %), whereas 70 patients (21.7 %) had a central venous catheter (CVC). Patients using CVC as a vascular access presented a decrease in four SF-36 domain scores, namely, physical functioning, emotional well-being, role-emotional, and energy/fatigue when compared with those using AVF as a vascular access. Additionally, these patients also showed significant decline in cognitive function and quality-of-social interaction domains. Left-arm AVF was associated with higher scores in three SF-36 domain scores, namely, physical functioning, pain, and general health. It was also associated with a higher score in ESRD target areas of symptoms/problem list and effects of kidney disease and quality-of-social interaction domains. The authors concluded that ESRD patients under OL-HDF using AVF as a vascular access had higher HRQOL scores in several domains when compared with those using CVC. Patients using AVF in the left forearm presented with higher HRQOL scores [43].

4.13. Lin et al.

Lin et al. compared OL-HDF (thrice, twice, and once per week) with different frequencies of combination high-flux HD. Interdialytic symptomatic hypotensive episodes were reduced when frequencies of online HDF were increased. Interdialysis physical well-being and symptoms similarly improved when frequency of HDF is increased to three times per week [44].

http://dx.doi.org/10.5772/64591

4.14. Nistor I et al.

Nistor et al. [45] conducted a systematic review of randomized controlled trials in which data for quality of life were extractable from eight trials (988 participants), including six evaluating HDF and one each evaluating HF or acetate-free biofiltration [33, 34, 36, 39–42, 44]. The authors Stated that in very low-quality evidence, data for quality of life were inconsistent. Data from the four parallel-group trials [33, 36, 39, 41] showed that there was no difference in the change in quality of life (any domain) comparing HDF with HD in one trial [36]. Both HDF and HD patients reported significant improvement in physical symptoms irrespective of treatment allocation in a second trial [41]. Hemodialysis patients had lower physical well-being scores than patients on HDF, but treatment effects on work tolerance and mental alertness were not available in a third trial [33]. Comparative data for HF and HD were not available in a fourth trial [39]. The remaining four studies were crossover design, and data for the end of the first phase of treatment were not available.

5. Summary

The available data on HRQOL in patients under OL-HDF therapy is limited and of low quality. Most parallel-group randomized clinical trials on this subject demonstrate no or limited improvement in HRQOL associated with OL-HDF. However, several crossover studies support a beneficial role of OL-HDF in enhancing quality of life in these patients. The effect of online HDF on quality of life reported by clinical studies is variable. The inconsistency of these results is probably related to different methods used to assess quality of life, sample size, duration of study, and the different characteristics of the convective therapy utilized such as blood flow rate, vascular access type and type of the dialyzer, convection volume, and frequency of online HDF. The most widely used and tested method of assessing health-related quality of life in patients undergoing online HDF replacement therapy is Kidney Disease Quality of Life Short Form-36 (KDQOL-SF-36). It is easily administrable and has been validated.

With the increased popularity of OL-HDF as a renal replacement therapy, larger better organized studies will probably become available in the future. Such studies, hopefully, will better clarify the issue.

Author details

Samir H. Almueilo

Address all correspondence to: smueilo@uod.edu.sa

King Fahd Hospital of the University, University of Dammam, Alkhobar, Saudi Arabia

References

[1] Collins AJ, Foley RN, Chavers B. United States Renal Data System 2011 annual data report: atlas of chronic kidney disease and end-stage renal disease in the United States. Am J Kidney Dis 2012; 59(1 suppl. 1):e1–e420

[2] Cheung AK, Rocco MV, Yan G, Leypoldt JK, Levin NW, Greene T, Agodoa L, Bailey J, Beck GJ, Clark W, Levey AS, Ornt DB, Schulman G, Schwab S, Teehan B, Eknoyan G. Serum beta-2 microglobulin levels predict mortality in dialysis patients: results of the HEMO study. J Am Soc Nephrol 2006; 17:546–555

[3] Canaud B, Bragg-Gresham JL, Marshall MR, Desmeules S, Gillespie BW, Depner T, Klassen P, Port FK. Mortality risk for patients receiving hemodiafiltration versus hemodialysis: European results from the DOPPS. Kidney Int. 2006; 69(11):2087–2093.

[4] Grooteman MP, van den Dorpel MA, Bots ML, Penne EL, van der Weerd NC, Mazairac AH, den Hoedt CH, van der Tweel I, Lévesque R, Nubé MJ, ter Wee PM, Blankestijn PJ, CONTRAST Investigators. Effect of online hemodiafiltration on all-cause mortality and cardiovascular outcomes. J Am Soc Nephrol 2012; 23:1087–1096

[5] Ok E, Asci G, Toz H, Ok ES, Kircelli F, Yilmaz M, Hur E, Demirci MS, Demirci C, Duman S, Basci A, Adam SM, Isik IO, Zengin M, Suleymanlar G, Yilmaz ME, Ozkahya M, Turkish Online Haemodiafiltration Study. Mortality and cardiovascular events in online haemodiafiltration (OL-HDF) compared with high-flux dialysis: results from the Turkish OL-HDF Study. Nephrol Dial Transplant 2013; 28:192–202

[6] Maduell F, Moreso F, Pons M, Ramos R, Mora-Macià J, Carreras J, Soler J, Torres F, Campistol JM, Martinez-Castelao A, ESHOL Study Group. High-efficiency postdilution online hemodiafiltration reduces all-cause mortality in hemodialysis patients. J Am Soc Nephrol 2013; 24:487–497

[7] Mercadal L, Franck JE, Metzger M, Urena Torres P, de Cornelissen F, Edet S, Béchade C, Vigneau C, Drueke T, Jacquelinet C, Stengel B, REIN Registry. Hemodiafiltration Versus Hemodialysis and Survival in Patients With ESRD: The French Renal Epidemiology and Information Network (REIN) Registry. Am J Kidney Dis 2015 Dec 24. pii: S0272-6386(15)01436-5. doi: 10.1053/j.ajkd.2015.11.016. [Epub ahead of print]

[8] Canaud B, Bragg-Gresham JL, Marshall MR, Desmeules S, Gillespie BW, Depner T, Klassen P, Port FK. Mortality risk for patients receiving hemodiafiltration versus hemodialysis: European results from the DOPPS. Kidney Int 2006; 69:2087–2093

[9] Mapes DL, Lopes AA, Satayathum S, McCullough KP, Goodkin DA, Locatelli F, Fukuhara S, Young EW, Kurokawa K, Saito A, Bommer J, Wolfe RA, Held PJ, Port FK et al. Health-related quality of life as a predictor of mortality and hospitalization: the Dialysis Outcomes and Practice Patterns Study (DOPPS). Kidney Int 2003; 64:339–349

[10] World Health Organization. Preamble to the Constitution of the World Health Organization as adopted by the International Health Conference, New York, 19–22 June, 1946.

In: Constitution of the World Health Organization, Geneva, Switzerland, World Health Organization, 1948, p 100

[11] The WHOQOL Group. The World Health Organization Quality of Life Assessment (WHOQOL). Development and psychometric properties. Soc Sci Med 1998;46:1569–1585

[12] Constitution of the World Health Organization. World Health Organization. Handbook of basic documents, 5th ed. Geneva: Palais des Nations, 1952:3–20, www.who.int/msa/qol/ql1.htm

[13] DeOreo PB. Hemodialysis patient-assessed functional health status predicts continued survival, hospitalization, and dialysis-attendance compliance. Am J Kidney Dis 1997;30:204–212.

[14] Ifudu O, Paul HR, Homel P, Friedman EA . Predictive value of functional status for mortality in patients on maintenance hemodialysis. Am J Nephrol 1998;18:109–116

[15] Gandek B, Sinclair SJ, Kosinski M, Ware JE Jr. Psychometric evaluation of the SF-36 health survey in Medicare managed care. Health Care Financ Rev 2004;25(4):5–25.

[16] McHorney CA. Health status assessment methods for adults: past accomplishments and future directions. Annu Rev Public Health 1999; 20:309–335.

[17] Selim AJ, Rogers W, Fleishman JA, Qian SX, Fincke BG, Rothendler JA, Kazis LE. Updated U.S. population standard for the Veterans RAND 12-item Health Survey (VR-12). Qual Life Res 2009;18(1):43–52.

[18] Testa MA, Simonson DC . Assessment of quality-of-life outcomes. N Engl J Med 1996;334:835–840

[19] Edgell ET, Coons SJ, Carter WB, Kallich JD, Mapes D, Damush TM, Hays RD. A review of health-related quality-of-life measures used in end-stage renal disease. Clin Ther 1996;18:887–938.

[20] Hays RD, Kallich JD, Mapes DL, Coons SJ, Carter WB. Development of the Kidney Disease Quality of Life (KDQOL) instrument. Qual Life Res 1994; 3: 329–338.

[21] Hays RD, Kallich JD, Mapes DL. Kidney Dialysis Quality of Life Short Form (KDQOL-SF) Version 1.3: A Manual for Use and Scoring. Santa Monica, CA: RAND, 1997.

[22] Mapes DL, Bragg-Gresham JL, Bommer J, Fukuhara S, McKevitt P, Wikstrom B, Lopes AA. Health-related quality of life in the Dialysis Outcomes and Practice Patterns Study (DOPPS). Am J Kidney Dis 2004; 44(suppl 2):54–60.

[23] Unruh M, Benz R, Greene T, Yan G, Beddhu S, DeVita M, Dwyer JT, Kimmel PL, Kusek JW, Martin A, Rehm-McGillicuddy J, Teehan BP, Meyer KB. Effects of hemodialysis dose and membrane flux on health-related quality of life in the HEMO Study. Kidney Int 2004; 66:355–366.

[24] Manns B, Johnson JA, Taub K, Mortis G, Ghali WA, Donaldson C. Quality of life in patients treated with hemodialysis or peritoneal dialysis: what are the important determinants? Clin Nephrol 2003; 60: 341–351.

[25] Ware JE, Snow KK, Kosinski M, Gandek B. SF-36 Health Survey-Manual and Interpretation Guide. Boston: The Health Institute, New England Medical Center, 1993

[26] Laupacis A, Muirhead N, Keown P, Wong C. A disease specific questionnaire for assessing quality of life in patients on hemodialysis. Nephron 1992; 60: 302–303

[27] The EuroQol Group. EuroQol—a new facility for the measurement of health-related quality of life. Health Policy 1990;16(3):199–208

[28] Wu AW, Fink NE, Cagney KA, Bass EB, Rubin HR, Meyer KB, Sadler JH, Powe NR. Developing a health-related quality-of-life measure for end-stage renal disease: the CHOICE Health Experience Questionnaire. Am J Kidney Dis 2001;37(1):11–21.

[29] Powe NR, Klag MJ, Sadler JH, Anderson GF, Bass EB, Briggs WA, Fink NE, Levey AS, Levin NW, Meyer KB, Rubin HR, Wu AW. Choices for healthy outcomes in caring for end-stage renal disease. Semin Dial 1996; 9:9–11.

[30] Moura A, Madureira J, Alija P, Fernandes JC, Oliveira JG, Lopez M, Filgueiras M, Amado L, Sameiro-Faria M, Miranda V, Mesquita E, Santos-Silva A, Costa E. Predictors of health-related quality of life perceived by end-stage renal disease patients under online hemodiafiltration. Qual Life Res (2015) 24:1327–1335

[31] Knezevic MZ, Djordjevic VV, Radovanovic-Velickovic RM, Stankovic JJ, Cvetkovic TP, Djordjevic VM. Influence of dialysis modality and membrane flux on quality of life in hemodialysis patients. Ren Fail 2012; 34(7):849–855

[32] Karkar A, Abdelrahman M, Locatelli F. A randomized trial on health-related patient satisfaction level with high-efficiency online hemodiafiltration versus high-flux dialysis. Blood Purif 2015;40:84–91

[33] Kantartzi K, Panagoutsos S, Mourvati E, Roumeliotis A, Leivaditis K, Devetzis V, Passadakis P, Vargemezis V. Can dialysis modality influence quality of life in chronic hemodialysis patients? Low-flux hemodialysis versus high-flux hemodiafiltration: a cross-over study. Ren Fail 2013;35(2):216–221.

[34] Schiffl H. Prospective randomized cross-over long-term comparison of online haemodiafiltration and ultrapure high-flux haemodialysis. Eur J Med Res 2007; 12:26–33

[35] Penne EL, Blankestijn PJ, Bots ML, van den Dorpel MA, Grooteman MP, Nube MJ, van der Tweel I, Ter Wee PM, the CONTRAST study group. Effect of increased convective clearance by on-line hemodiafiltration on all cause and cardiovascular mortality in chronic hemodialysis patients—the Dutch CONvective TRAnsport STudy (CONTRAST): Rationale and design of a randomised controlled trial [ISRCTN38365125]. Curr Control Trials Cardiovasc Med 2005; 6:8

[36] Grooteman MP, van den Dorpel MA, Bots ML, Penne EL, van der Weerd NC, Mazairac AH, den Hoedt CH, van der Tweel I, Lévesque R, Nubé MJ, ter Wee PM, Blankestijn PJ, CONTRAST Investigators. Effect of online hemodiafiltration on all-cause mortality and cardiovascular outcomes. J Am Soc Nephrol 2012; 23:1087–1096

[37] Mazairac AH, de Wit GA, Grooteman MP, Penne EL, van der Weerd NC, den Hoedt CH, Lévesque R, van den Dorpel MA, Nubé MJ, ter Wee PM, Bots ML, Blankestijn PJ, CONTRAST Investigators. Effect of hemodiafiltration on quality of life over time. Clin J Am Soc Nephrol 2013;8(1):82–89

[38] Moura A, Madureira J, Alija P, Fernandes JC, Oliveira JG, Lopez M, Filgueiras M, Amado L, Sameiro-Faria M, Miranda V, Santos-Silva A, Costa E. Effect of aging in the perception of health-related quality of life in end-stage renal disease patients under online-hemodiafiltration. Aging Dis 2015;6(1):17–26

[39] Beerenhout CH, Luik AJ, Jeuken-Mertens SG, Bekers O, Menheere P, Hover L, Klaassen L, van der Sande FM, Cheriex EC, Meert N, Leunissen KM, Kooman JP. Pre-dilution on-line haemofiltration vs low-flux haemodialysis: a randomized prospective study. Nephrol Dial Transplant 2005;20(6):1155–1163

[40] Stefánsson BV, Abramson M, Nilsson U, Haraldsson B. Hemodiafiltration improves plasma 25-hepcidin levels: a prospective, randomized, blinded, cross-over study comparing hemodialysis and hemodiafiltration. Nephron Extra 2012;2:55–65

[41] Ward RA, Schmidt B, Hullin J, Hillebrand GF, Samtleben W. A comparison of on-line hemodiafiltration and high-flux hemodialysis: a prospective clinical study. J Am Soc Nephrol 2000;11(12):2344–2350.

[42] Verzetti G, Navino C,Bolzani R, Galli G, Panzetta G. Acetate-free biofiltration versus bicarbonate haemodialysis in the treatment of patients with diabetic nephropathy: a cross-over multicentric study. Nephrol Dial Transplant 1998; 13:955–961

[43] Moura A, Madureira J, Alija P, Fernandes JC, Oliveira JG, Lopez M, Filgueiras M, Amado L, Sameiro-Faria M, Miranda V, Vieira M, Santos-Silva A, Costa E. Type of vascular access and location in online hemodiafiltration and its association with patient's perception of health-related quality of life. J Vasc Access 2014; 15(3):175–182

[44] Lin CL, Huang CC, Chang CT, Wu MS, Hung CC, Chien CC, Yang CW. Clinical improvement by increased frequency of on-line hemodialfiltration. Ren Fail 2001; 23(2): 193–206.

[45] Nistor I, Palmer SC, Craig JC, Saglimbene V, Vecchio M, Covic A, Strippoli GF. Convective versus diffusive dialysis therapies for chronic kidney failure: an updated systematic review of randomized controlled trials. Am J Kidney Dis 2014; 63(6):954–967

Chapter 9

Cost-Effectiveness of Online Hemodiafiltration

Khalid AlSaran and Khalid Mirza

Additional information is available at the end of the chapter

http://dx.doi.org/10.5772/64679

Abstract

Care of patients with end-stage renal disease (ESRD) is essential but also resource intense. We review several studies on online hemodiafiltration (OL-HDF), which concluded that high-volume OL-HDF is associated with better outcome compared to conventional hemodialysis. The cost-effectiveness of OL-HDF was shown in many studies. For example, in the Canadian setting of the Convective Transport Study (CONTRAST), the high-efficiency OL-HDF was shown to be cost-effective compared with low-flux hemodialysis (LF-HD) for patients with ESRD. In our study (Al Saran et al.), it was shown that the cost of hemodialysis was quite less in Saudi Arabia than in other industrialized countries while maintaining a high standard of care. In our retrospective analysis of the cost of OL-HDF in the same center, it was only 3% higher than the conventional HD, which indicates that it is cost-effective considering the improved hospitalization rate, the mortality rates, and the likely better quality of life associated with it. The trend of increased practice of OL-HDF may encourage the practice of home OL-HDF as well. It has been shown that home HD is more cost-effective than in-center HD and we presume that the same results will be applied to home OL-HDF as well.

Keywords: online hemodiafiltration, low-flux hemodialysis, middle molecules, cost

1. Introduction

Untreated end-stage renal disease (ESRD) carries a high mortality. The management of ESRD is either by dialysis or by a kidney transplant. Due to insufficient number of kidney donors in comparison with the progressive increase in the number of ESRD patients in need for dialysis,

dialysis remains the main modality of treatment. Since the care of patients with ESRD is resource intense, it is necessary to adopt measures that render the delivery of dialysis more cost-effective and improve the quality of care. The uremic syndrome is characterized by the accumulation of uremic toxins due to inadequate kidney function. The European Uremic Toxin Work Group has listed more than 90 compounds considered to be uremic toxins. Among them, 68 have a molecular weight less than 500 Da, 10 have between 500 and 12,000 Da, and 12 exceed 12,000 Da [1]. Solutes weighing less than 500 Da are considered low molecular weight solutes and they are removed by passive diffusion down a favorable concentration gradient. Urea is considered a marker of such toxins. Its clearance, as measured by Kt/V urea, correlates with patient morbidity showing the evidence that such toxins contribute to the uremic syndrome [2]. The mortality rate of patient on maintenance dialysis has been found to be 15–20% [3]. This is despite improvements in patient care and technology. In order to increase survival in dialysis patients, it was postulated in 1983 that increasing the Kt/V in conventional dialysis may help to reduce mortality. However, the hemodialysis (HEMO) study failed to show a positive effect on patient survival when dialysis dose per hemodialysis session was increased above the current K/DOQI recommendations [4]. Possible explanation for this unfavorable outcome could be in the kinetics of urea removal which is representative of small solutes, but not of larger-sized molecules such as middle molecules, large molecular weight proteins or protein-bound solutes, thereby making Kt/V misleading [5]. Clearance of urea accounts for only one-sixth of physiological clearance [1]. In addition, several shortcomings are associated with short dialysis schedules that are not captured by Kt/V index such as extracellular fluid volume control, phosphate control, and adequate removal of middle and larger uremic molecules compounds. Beta-2 microglobulin levels are associated with the development of dialysis-related amyloidosis and possibly reduced survival [6]. It seems likely that beta-2 microglobulin is a marker for overall-middle molecule clearance, including more toxic and yet unidentified uremic compounds [7–10]. Those solutes are better removed by high-flux membranes due to their more porous characteristics with increased permeability. Hemodialfiltration (HDF) is the treatment modality that combines diffusion and enhanced convection in order to facilitate removal of small molecular weight solutes. Moreover, small molecule removal is further increased with the use of high-volume OL-HDF. HDF is thus a more cardioprotective renal replacement therapy.

Recent randomized controlled trials (RCTs) have shown the survival advantage of HDF using high-convective volumes (23 L/session or 69 L/week prescription). In Peters et al.'s review [11] which is a pooled individual participant analysis of 4 RCTs, it was a observed that in patients receiving the higher delivered convection volume (>23 L per 1.73 m^2 body surface area (BSA) per session), the longest survival benefit was seen with **Hazard Ratio (HR)** of 0.69 (95% CI: 0.47; 1.00) for cardiovascular disease mortality and HR of 0.78 (95% CI: 0.62; 0.98) for all-cause mortality.

In another study by Canaud et al. [12], which was a retrospective data collection from over 2000 patients with a minimum follow-up of 2 years, the relative survival rate of OL-HDF patients was found to increase at about 55 **L**–75 **L**/week of convection volume.

http://dx.doi.org/10.5772/64679

2. Principles of hemodiafiltration

Ultrafiltrate volume is removed by the dialysis machine through increased transmembrane pressure (TMP), whereas the replacement solution is infused intravenously at equal volume minus the desired fluid volume removal to preserve extracellular fluid balance and isovolemic state. The replaced solution represents *substitution volume,* whereas convective volume represents the sum of substitution volume and desired fluid volume removal during the dialysis session. The fluid can be substituted either after the **dialyser** as the reference mode (post-dilution mode) or before the **dialyser** (pre-dilution mode) or the combination of both (mixed dilution mode).

3. Efficacy of online hemodiafiltration

Several studies have shown online hemodiafiltration (OL-HDF) to be superior to conventional hemodialysis in reducing all-cause mortality in hemodialysis patients. OL-HDF has been found to reduce cardiovascular events as compared with conventional hemodialysis.

Furthermore, OL-HDF has significantly improved patients' satisfaction and quality of life [13–16]. OL-HDF has also shown to be a cost-effective treatment for ESRD [17]. For example, in the prospective Convective Transport Study (CONTRAST), there was no significant difference between treatment groups with regard to all-cause mortality (121 versus 127 deaths per 1000 person-years in the OL-HDF and LF-HD groups, respectively); (hazard ratio, 0.95; 95% confidence interval, 0.75–1.20) after a mean follow-up of 3 years (range 0.4–6.6 years). Receiving high-volume hemodiafiltration during the trial was associated with lower all-cause mortality.

In the ESHOL multicentre, open-label RCT [14], patients on OL-HDF compared with those on HD had a 55% lower risk of infection-related mortality (HR, 0.45; 95% CI, 0.21–0.96; $P = 0.03$), a 33% lower risk of cardiovascular mortality (HR, 0.67; 95% CI, 0.44–1.02; $P = 0.06$), and a 30% lower risk of all-cause mortality (**HR**, 0.70; 95% confidence interval [95% CI], 0.53–0.92; P = 0.01). In conclusion, high-efficiency post-dilution OL-HDF reduces all-cause mortality compared with conventional hemodialysis. According to the Turkish OL-HF prospective RCT [15], 782 patients undergoing thrice-weekly HD were enrolled and randomly assigned in a 1:1 ratio to either postdilution OL-HDF or high-flux HD. Using a filtration volume of 17.2 ± 1.3 **L, there** was no difference in the primary outcome between the two groups (event-free survival of 77.6% in OL-HDF vs. 74.8% in the high-flux group, $P = 0.28$). Also, no difference was seen in the cardiovascular and overall survival, number of hypotensive episodes and hospitalization rate. However on further analysis, the patients who received higher substitution volume (>17.4 L per session) had better cardiovascular outcome ($P = 0.002$) and overall survival ($P = 0.03$) compared with those who received high-flux HD. The study of Karkar et al. [16] aimed to investigate the effect of OL-HDF versus high-flux HD (HF) on a patient's health-related satisfaction level. A higher satisfaction level was achieved by the OL-HDF group compared with HF group ($p < 0.0001$). In the OL-HDF group, there was less itching (9 ± 10 vs.

48 ± 10), less cramps (3 ± 5 vs. 55 ± 8), less joint pain and stiffness (24 ± 10 vs. 83 ± 8) with improvement in sexual performance (57 ± 10 vs. 5 ± 5), social activity (82 ± 9 vs. 15 ± 8), and general mood (94 ± 9 vs. 28 ± 16). High-efficiency postdilution online HDF versus high-flux HD significantly improved patients' satisfaction and quality of life, including social, physical, and professional activities.

4. Cost-effectiveness of OL-HDF

4.1. Review of the literature

In spite of the several studies which investigate the efficacy of OL-HDF, there were fewer studies which assessed the cost-effectiveness of this procedure. One of them was the CONTRAST [17] in which the cost-effectiveness of high-efficiency OL-HDF was compared with LF-HD for patients with ESRD based on the Canadian (Centre Hospitalier de l'Universite de Montreal) arm of a parallel-group RCT. Over a period of 74 months, an economic evaluation was conducted. To simulate costs and health benefits over lifetime, a Markov state transition model was constructed. A total of 130 patients were randomly allocated to OL-HDF (n = 67) and LF-HD (n = 63). The primary outcome was costs per quality-adjusted life-year (QALY) gained. The cost-utility ratio of OL-HDF versus LF-HD was Can$53,270 per QALY gained over lifetime, and it was fairly robust in the sensitivity analysis. It was concluded that in a Canadian setting, high-efficiency OL-HDF can be considered as a cost-effective treatment for ESRD.

In Mazairac et al. study [18], a cost-utility analysis was performed using a Markov model. It included data from the CONTRAST. Probabilistic sensitivity analyses were performed to study uncertainty, and costs were estimated using a societal perspective. Total annual costs for HDF and HD were €88,622 ± 19,272 and €86,086 ± 15,945, respectively (in 2009 euros). The incremental cost per quality-adjusted life year (QALY) of HDF versus HD was €287,679 when modeled over a 5-year period. Even under the most favorable assumptions like a high-convection volume (>20.3 L), this amount will not fall below €140,000 using sensitivity analyses. They concluded that HDF cannot be considered a cost-effective treatment for patients with end-stage renal disease at present. This was based on accepted societal willingness-to-pay thresholds.

Various factors may responsible for the true differences in the cost of dialysis provision between various studies. These factors may include variable standards of care, different management protocols, differences in the methodologies used, the older population of patients with more comorbid illness (especially in the United States), different import duties and shipping charges, local labor costs, dates of the studies, the differences in countries in which the analyses were carried out, nurse/patient and physician/patient ratios and the number of dialysis sessions. Direct comparisons may not be very informative. Finally, the comparison between countries in the cost of dialysis must take into consideration the morbidity and mortality outcomes in these patients, as well as perceived quality of life [19, 20].

We have previously [21] assessed the cost of hemodialysis according to the treatment protocols based on the current Kidney Disease Outcome Quality Initiative (K/DOQI) guidelines. The cost data, which included direct and overhead costs, were analyzed during the period from 1 January 2007 to 30 June 2010. Direct cost included items related to dialysis treatment such as dialysis disposables, dialysis related drugs, medical personnel, outpatient medications, laboratory, and other ancillary survives.

The category	The cost/session		Percentage
(I) Direct cost	USD	SR	
(1) Dialysis disposables (including tubing, dialyzer, acid concentrate, needles, normal saline, dressing set, heparin and bed sheets)	40.53	152	13.64
(2) Medical equipments and maintenance	13.6	51	4.58
(3) The meals	7.12	26.7	2.40
(4) Personnel:			
a. Administrative	32	120	10.77
b. Medical	90.13	338	30.34
(5) Intravenous medications			
a. ESA	16.8	63	5.66
b. Vitamin D	1.06	4	0.36
c. Iron	0.8	3	0.27
d. Albumin and dextrose	0.53	2	0.18
(6) Vascular access creation and revision*	10.24	38.4	3.45
(7) Laboratory tests	10.19	38.2	3.43
(8) Imaging investigations	0.11	0.7	0.06
(9) Out-patient and crash cart medications	17.87	67	6
Total direct cost	241	904	81.15
(II) Indirect cost			
(1) Non-medical equipments with maintenance and housekeeping	15.55	58.3	5.23
(2) Medical records	0.5	1.86	0.17
(3) Building**	29	109	9.78
(4) Disposal of medical waste	0.71	2.66	0.24
(5) Meals for personnel	7.12	26.7	2.40
(6) Suit for personnel	0.22	0.83	0.07
(7) Automobile maintenance and fuel	1.28	4.8	0.43
(8) Utility bills (electricity, water and phone)	1.56	5.85	0.53
Total indirect cost	56	210	18.85
Total	297	1114	100

*Calculated based on the mean half-life of the access and on the mean frequency rate of re-insertion or revision.
**Calculated based on the current cost for the land and construction divided by 20 years for the construction and by 10 years for the land (investment rate).

Table 1. The unit cost of the categories associated with hemodialysis provision at the King Salman Center for kidney diseases.

Over head (indirect) cost included building, maintenance and engineering costs, housekeeping and administrative personnel. The mean total cost per HD session was calculated as 297 US dollars (USD) [1114 Saudi Riyals (SR)], and the mean total cost of dialysis per patient per year was 46,332 USD (173,784 SR). Out of the total cost, the direct cost was the major part (81.15%) (**Table 1**). The total cost was well below the average cost in the industrialized countries although a high standard of care was maintained.

The category	Hemodialysis	Hemodiafiltration
(I) Direct cost		
(1) Dialysis disposables (include tubing, dialyzer, acid concentrate, needles, normal saline, dressing set, heparin and bed sheets)	40.53	50.53
(2) Medical equipments and maintenance	13.6	13.6
(3) The meals	7.12	7.12
(4) Personnel		
a. Administrative	32	32
b. Medical	90.13	90.13
(5) Intravenous medications		
a. ESA	16.8	16.8
b. Vitamin D	1.06	1.06
c. Iron	0.8	0.8
d. Albumin and dextrose	0.53	0.53
(6) Vascular access creation and revision	10.24	10.24
(7) Laboratory tests	10.19	10.19
(8) Imaging investigations	0.11	0.11
(9) Out-patient and crash cart medications	17.87	17.87
Total direct cost	241	251
(II) Indirect cost		
(1) Nonmedical equipments with maintenance and housekeeping	15.55	15.55
(2) Medical records	0.5	0.5
(3) Building**	29	29
(4) Disposal of medical waste	0.71	0.71
(5) Meals for personnel	7.12	7.12
(6) Suit for personnel	0.22	0.22
(7) Automobile maintenance and fuel	1.28	1.28
(8) Utility bills (electricity, water, and phone)	1.56	1.56
Total indirect cost	56	56
Total	297	307

Table 2. Comparison of the cost/session between hemodialysis and hemodiafiltration in US dollar.

4.2. Retrospective comparison between HD and OL-HDF

In our retrospective analysis of the cost of OL-HDF in the same center, the cost of the OL-HDF was only 3.4% higher than the conventional HD (10 US dollar difference per session). This difference in cost was in the category of dialysis disposables (**Table 2**). It is attributed to (1) the cost of the water purification filter at the back of online HDF dialysis machine which cost an average of 1.95 USD/session, (2) the cost of tubing extension used for OL-HDF which cost 7.8 USD/session, (3) the cost of the treated water used as substitution fluid (its volume in our center was 30 L/session), which cost 0.25 USD/session. This little difference in the cost of water treatment between the two modalities may be attributed to the fact that we are using ultrapure water for the two modalities in order to minimize the risk of micro-inflammation associated with HD. We need to emphasize that in some centers that have the latest manufactured dialysis machine, there will be no extra cost for the tubing as it will be the same tubing in both modalities. Finally, there was no difference in the cost for using high-flux dialyzer as its price nowadays is almost the same as for low-flux dialyzer. In conclusion, this minor cost difference between HD and OL-HDF indicates that OL-HDF is cost-effective considering the advantages of the OL-HDF and the better quality of life associated with it. The possible presumed decrease in the cost of medications and hospitalization is another supportive factor for the cost-effectiveness of OL-HDF. In addition, OL-HDF may not be indicated for all the dialysis patients. In our center, OL-HDF was only performed for certain indications such as severe hyperphosphatemia, severe resistant hypertension, and resistant anemia.

4.3. The cost-effectiveness of home HD and home OL-HDF

The trend of increased practice of OL-HDF may encourage the practice of home OL-HDF as well. More intensive and/or frequent hemodialysis may provide clinical benefits to patients with ESRD; however, these dialysis treatments are more convenient to the patients if provided in their homes. It has been shown that home HD is more cost-effective than in-center HD, and we presume that the same results will be applied to home OL-HDF as well. In Komenda et al. [22] review of data from Australia, Canada, and the United Kingdom, it was noted that the cost of the first year for all hemodialysis modalities were higher than in subsequent years, and the cost for conventional home hemodialysis was lower than in-center hemodialysis in subsequent years. Their conclusions were similar to previous studies that home-based conventional and more frequent hemodialysis may provide clinical benefit at reasonable costs. In another study for Komenda et al. [23], they described a comprehensive funding model for a large centrally administered but locally delivered home hemodialysis program in British Columbia, Canada. There were 122 patients, of which 113 were still in the program at study end. In this two-year retrospective study, the majority of patients performed home nocturnal hemodialysis, and it was found that the total cost for home hemodialysis was higher in the first two years and it was lower by about 10,500 per year in the subsequent years. So their study explained a valid, comprehensive funding model delineating reliable cost estimates of starting as well as maintaining a large home-based hemodialysis program. Therefore, when designing budgets for home hemodialysis, consideration of hidden costs is important for administrators and planners.

McFarlane et al. [24] assessed the cost-effectiveness of home nocturnal hemodialysis (HNHD) in relative to in-center hemodialysis (IHD). In this Canadian one-year prospective study which was done at two centers in Toronto in the year 2000, HNHD had a higher mean number of treatments per week (5.7 vs. 3.0, $P = 0.004$). In the cost categories, staffing was found to be less expensive for HNHD (weekly $210 vs. $423, $P < 0.001$, PMA $4179 vs. $12,393). There was a trend toward lower costs for hospital procedures and admissions (weekly $23 vs. $134, $P = 0.355$, PMA $1173 vs. $6997), for the capital costs (weekly $118 vs. $17, $P < 0.001$, PMA $6139 vs. $871) and the cost of direct hemodialysis materials (weekly $318 vs. $126, $P < 0.001$, PMA $16,587 vs. $6575). On the other hand, there was a trend toward higher cost for laboratory tests (weekly $33 vs. $26, $P = 0.094$, PMA $1744 vs. $1364). Physician costs were the same at $128 per week (PMA $6650). The projected mean annual costs were more than $10,000 lower ($56,394 vs. $68,935). The weekly mean total cost for health care delivery was 20% less for HNHD ($1082 vs. $1322, $P = 0.006$). Their conclusion was that HNHD provides about three times as many treatment hours at nearly a one-fifth lower cost. The savings were evident even when only program and funding specific costs were considered.

5. Conclusion

OL-HDF seems to be cost-effective and much better than conventional hemodialysis for the patient's satisfaction, quality of life, patient's survival, dialysis-related mortality and morbidity, and cardiovascular outcomes. However, more prospective studies are needed on the cost-effectiveness of this procedure.

Acknowledgements

The authors are grateful to Engineer Fahad Alderh for his contribution in cost calculation.

Author details

Khalid AlSaran[1,2,3*] and Khalid Mirza[4]

*Address all correspondence to: Khalid_aln@yahoo.co.uk

1 Pediatric Nephrology Department, King Saud Medical City, Riyadh, Saudi Arabia

2 College of Medicine, Alfaisal University, Riyadh, Saudi Arabia

3 King Salman Kidney Center, Riyadh, Saudi Arabia

4 King Saud Medical City, Riyadh, Saudi Arabia

References

[1] Yavuz, A., et al, *Uremic toxins: a new focus on an old subject*. Semin Dial, 2005. 18(3): pp. 203–11

[2] Lowrie EG, Laird NM, Henry RR: Protocol for the National Cooperative Dialysis Study. *Kidney Int* 23(Suppl 13):S11–S18, 1983.

[3] System: U.T.U.S.R.D, *Overall hospitalization and mortality*. Am J Kidney Dis, 2010. 55(Suppl 1): p. S1

[4] Lowrie, E.G., N.M. Laird and R.R. Henry, *Protocol for the National Cooperative Dialysis Study*. Kidney Int Suppl, 1983. (13): pp. S11–8

[5] Ejnoyan, G., et al, *Effect of dialysis dose and membrane flux in maintenance hemodialysis*. N Engl J Med 2002. 347(25): pp. 2010–9

[6] Winchester, J.F., J.A. Salsberg and N.W. Levin, *Beta-2 microglobulin in ESRD*: an in-depth review. Adv Ren Replace Ther, 2003. 10(4): pp. 279–309

[7] National Kidney Foundation, K/DOQl clinical practice guidelines for bone metabolism and disease in chronic kidney disease. Am J Kidney Dis, 2003. 42(4 Suppl 3):S1–201.

[8] Gejyo, F., et al, *Beta 2-microglobulin: a new form of amyloid protein associated with chronic hemodialysis*. Kidney Int, 1986. 30(3): pp. 385–90

[9] Koch, K.M., *Dialysis-related amyloidosis*. Kidney Int, 1992. 41(5): pp. 1416–29

[10] Miyata, T., et al, *Beta-2 microglobulin in renal disease.* J Am Soc Nephrol, 1998. 9(9): pp. 1723–35

[11] Peters, S.A.E., M.L. Bots, B. Canaud, et al. *Haemodiafiltration and mortality in end-stage kidney disease patients: a pooled individual participant data analysis from four randomized controlled trials*. Nephrol Dial Transplant (2015) 0: 1–7

[12] Bernard Canaud, Carlo Barbieri, Daniele Marcelli et al. Optimal convection volume for improving patient outcomes in an international incident dialysis cohort treated with online hemodiafiltration., Kidney Int 2015; 88(5):1108–16

[13] Muriel, P.C., M.A. van den Dorpel, et al, *Effect of online hemodiafiltration on all-cause mortality and cardiovascular outcome*. J Am Soc Nephrol, 2012. 23: pp. 1087–1096

[14] Maduell, F., F. Moreso, et al, *High-efficiency postdilution online hemodiafiltration reduces all-cause mortality in hemodialysis patients*. J Am Soc Nephrol, 2013. 24: pp. 487–497

[15] Ercan, O.k., G. Asci, et al., *Mortality and cardiovascular events in online Hemodiafiltration (OL-HDF) compared to high-flux dialysis: results from Turkish OL-HDF study*. Nephrol Dial Transplant, 2013. 28: pp. 192–202

[16] Karkar, A., M. Abdelrahman, et al, *A randomized trial on health-related patient satisfaction level with high-efficiency online hemodiafiltration versus high-flux dialysis.* Blood Purif, 2015. 40: pp. 84–91

[17] Levesque, R., D. Marcelli, et al, *Cost-effectiveness analysis of high efficiency hemodiafiltration versus low-flux hemodialysis based on Canadian arm of CONTRAST study.* Appl Health Econ Health Policy. 2015, 13 (6): pp. 647–59.

[18] Albert H.A. Mazairac, Peter J. Blankestijn, Muriel P.C. Grooteman et al. The cost–utility of haemodiafiltration versus haemodialysis in the Convective Transport Study. Nephrol Dial Transplant (2013); 28(7) :1865–73.

[19] Roderick, P., T. Nicholson, A. Armitage, et al. *An evaluation of the costs, effectiveness and quality of renal replacement therapy provision in renal satellite units in England and Wales.* Health Technol Assess, 2005. 9: pp. 1–178

[20] De Vecchi, A.F., M. Dratwa and M.E. Wiedemann. *Healthcare systems and end-stage renal disease (ESRD) therapies an international review: costs and reimbursement/funding of ESRD therapies.* Nephrol Dial Transplant, 1999. 14(Suppl 6): pp. 31–41

[21] Khalid AlSaran, Alaa Sabry, The cost of Hemodialysis in a Large Saudi Hemodialysis Center. Saudi KidneyDis Transplant. 2012; 23(1):78–82.

[22] Komenda P., M.B. Gavaghan, S. Susan, et al., *An economic assessment model for in-center, conventional home, and more frequent home hemodialysis.* Kidney Int, 2012. 81: pp. 307–13

[23] Komenda, P., M. Copland, J. Makwana, et al. *The cost of starting and maintaining a large home hemodialysis program.* Kidney Int, 2010. 77: pp. 1039–45

[24] Philip A. McFarlane, Andreas Pierratos, et al. Cost savings of home nocturnal versus conventional in-center hemodialysis. Kidney Int 2002; 62:2216–2222.

[25] Icks A, Haastret B, Gandjour A, et al. Cost of dialysis: a regional population based analysis. Nephrol Dial Transplant 2010; 25 (5):1647–52.